Salvador Santana Silva Júnior

Diagnosis and determination of copper in goats and sheep

AF537182

Salvador Santana Silva Júnior

Diagnosis and determination of copper in goats and sheep

ScienciaScripts

Imprint
Any brand names and product names mentioned in this book are subject to trademark, brand or patent protection and are trademarks or registered trademarks of their respective holders. The use of brand names, product names, common names, trade names, product descriptions etc. even without a particular marking in this work is in no way to be construed to mean that such names may be regarded as unrestricted in respect of trademark and brand protection legislation and could thus be used by anyone.

Cover image: www.ingimage.com

This book is a translation from the original published under ISBN 978-613-9-67126-7.

Publisher:
Sciencia Scripts
is a trademark of
Dodo Books Indian Ocean Ltd. and OmniScriptum S.R.L publishing group

120 High Road, East Finchley, London, N2 9ED, United Kingdom
Str. Armeneasca 28/1, office 1, Chisinau MD-2012, Republic of Moldova, Europe
Printed at: see last page
ISBN: 978-620-8-10821-2

Copyright © Salvador Santana Silva Júnior
Copyright © 2024 Dodo Books Indian Ocean Ltd. and OmniScriptum S.R.L publishing group

SUMMARY

To my family

I dedicate

ACKNOWLEDGMENTS

To **God...** who gave me life.

To *my Family....* My wife Lorena, My son icaro

My parents, Salvador Santana Silva and Maria das Graças Paiva Silva, my siblings, Salmâria, Silvia and Gedeval, my nephews Neto, Bruno and Bia and all my family who, with great affection and support, have spared no effort to get me to this stage of my life. Without them, it wouldn't be possible.

To Professor Alexandre Coutinho Antonelli for his patient guidance and encouragement, which made it possible to complete this dissertation.

To my colleagues on the master's course who passed on the knowledge and concepts that led me to complete this dissertation.

To *all the teachers and staff at Univasf*

and the Postgraduate Board of Animal Science.

To my friends and colleagues from the Postgraduate course in Animal Science, Jair, Rodrigo, Douglas, Percivaldo and Felipe, and from the undergraduate course, Josemario, George and lara, and all the others who contributed directly and indirectly to the completion of this work.

A big hug to everyone!

'It doesn't matter whether animals are incapable of thinking or not. What matters is that they are capable of suffering"

Jeremy Bentham

SUMMARY

Goat and sheep farming has always been considered a subsistence activity in the northeast of Brazil. However, the production of these ruminants has expanded and the Northeast has 90% of the country's goat herd and 56.7% of the sheep herd, but with very low zootechnical indices, as they are hampered by nutritional and health deficiencies. Among the main causes of the herd's low productivity is inadequate quantity and quality of nutrition, especially during the dry season, when there is a drop in fodder production, associated with mineral deficiencies in the soil and vegetation. Reports of mineral deficiencies have been recorded in several states in the Northeast region, such as copper, cobalt, zinc, manganese and iron in the states of Maranhão, Piaui, Cearà, Sergipe and Bahia. Copper deficiency can occur due to a lower supply of this microelement in the diet or the occurrence of antagonizing elements that reduce its availability, such as sulphur, iron and molybdenum. Copper supplementation is necessary in areas proven to be deficient in this element to avoid the occurrence of enzootic ataxia in kids and lambs. In the Petrolina micro-region in Pernambuco, there are no reports of surveys to determine the profile of essential trace elements in the biological materials of goats and sheep. The aim was therefore to determine the occurrence and distribution of copper deficiency in the Petrolina micro-region in Pernambuco, and to establish whether the deficiency is primary or secondary, in order to subsequently recommend correct forms of supplementation. It was found that there is no copper deficiency when looking at the average liver copper levels, only occasional deficiencies. Zinc levels are within a normal range, while iron levels are higher in sheep and molybdenum levels are lower in goats. It was also found that ceruloplasmin activity is a good indicator of serum copper levels.

Keywords: Sheep. Goats. Microminerals. Copper.

INTRODUCTION

Brazil has undergone transformations in the goat farming scene, and the expansion of agribusiness in this productive sector, which evolved from subsistence farming, is proving to be a source of sustainable income for many rural properties. The market has been growing rapidly, demanding greater concern with health and production aspects. Goat and sheep breeding needs to be based on sustainable farming systems that can guarantee better health, reproductive and nutritional conditions for these animals, through the supply of quality food, the use of biosecurity measures and reliable diagnostic tests that are accessible to all producers, most of whom are family farmers.

The census carried out by the Brazilian Institute of Geography and Statistics (IBGE) in 2010 shows a sheep herd of 17,380,581 million heads and a goat herd of 9,312,784 million heads. The Northeast region has a total herd of 9,857,754 head of sheep and 8,418,898 head of goats, representing 56.7% and 90% of the national sheep and goat herd respectively, followed by the South (4,886,541 sheep and 343,325 goats) and the Midwest (1,268,175 sheep and 113,427 goats), making it the largest national producer of both species.

The state of Pernambuco has a herd of 1,622,511 sheep and 1,735,051 goats. This is one of the most representative activities for rural producers, especially in the state's agreste and sertâo regions, where the Petrolina micro-region is located. The main herd in the territory is sheep with 329,200 head, representing 22% of the state's total, followed by goats with 292,800 head, representing 17.9% of the state's goat herd (BRASIL, 2010).

Knowledge of domestic animal diseases in the different regions of Brazil is important for determining efficient forms of prophylaxis and control. Guedes et al (2007) diagnosed two outbreaks of enzootic ataxia in Patos and Sâo Sebastiâo do Umbuzeiro in Paraiba, a disease related to copper deficiency. Another outbreak had been diagnosed in 1998 in the same state, in the municipality of Campina Grande. The occurrence of the disease in three different municipalities in the semi-arid region of Paraiba suggests that hypocuprosis may be a frequent deficiency in the northeast. This disease was also diagnosed in the 1960s in sheep in the state of Piaui (TOKARNIA et al. 1966). Santos et al. (2006) diagnosed cases of the same disease in sheep and goats in the state of Pernambuco in 2001 and 2002, suggesting further research into the subject in other areas of the state.

TERRITORIAL CHARACTERIZATION

The Territory of the Sertao do Sao Francisco is geographically located in the northeast of Brazil, in the Semi-Arid region of Pernambuco. The region's main access routes are BR 407, BR 428 and BR 122, and it is made up of seven municipalities: Afrânio, Cabrobó, Dormentes, Lagoa Grande, Orocó, Petrolina and Santa Maria da Boa Vista, as shown in the map below, (Figure 1):

Figure 1 - Map of the Petrolina micro-region in Pernambuco

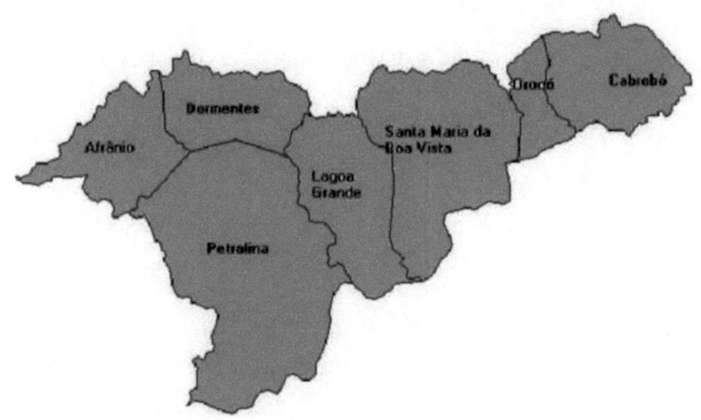

Source: SDT/MDA - 2011

The Territory of the Sertao do Sao Francisco covers an area of 14,682.2 km^2 , representing 14.89% of the total area of the State of Pernambuco, which is 98,588.3 km2, with Petrolina being the largest municipality, with 4,756.8 km2, covering approximately 32.4% of the total area of this territory. All the municipalities are located in the Mesoregion of Sao Francisco and in the Microregion of Petrolina. The territory's main potential and trademark is the River San Francisco. The proper and efficient management of water is the main lever for development in this territory, and most of the municipalities are the target of a set of public policies aimed at rural development (BRASIL, 2011).

literature review

1.1 THE IMPORTANCE OF COPPER IN THE BODY

The study of copper began in 1925 with Hart and collaborators, who discovered the importance of copper and iron in the formation of hemoglobin (MAYNARD, 1984). According to Davis and Mertz (1987 apud MONDAL; BISWAS, 2007), copper is an essential element for cattle and other animals to carry out a large number of biochemical functions.

The role and importance of copper in enzymatic systems in the metabolism of ruminants is well known. Copper has the peculiarity of being easily oxidized or reduced, a fundamental characteristic for the 26 copper metalloenzymes that catalyze oxidation-reduction reactions. Among the enzymes that depend directly on copper are: cytochrome oxidase, lysyl oxidase, tyrosinase, dopamine oxidase, urate oxidase, superoxide dismutase and butyryl-CoA dehydrogenase, among others (RIET-CORREA et al., 2006). It is also present in some metalloproteins such as ceruloplasmin, which regulates the activity of transferrin, and metallothionein, which, among other functions, regulates the absorption of copper itself by the body (ORTOLANI, 2002). In animals, it participates in the formation of myelin and bones, hematopoiesis, tissue binding metabolism, pigmentation and the formation of wool and hair (CAVALHEIRO; TRINDADE, 1992; RADOSTITS et al. 2007).

The excess or lack of copper, similar to other macro and micro elements, can cause both intoxication and deficiency in animals, respectively (SUTTLE, 2010). Hypocuprosis is one of the deficiencies of greatest interest in ruminants, showing various symptoms and cosmopolitan distribution, as it occurs both in our country and in other parts of the world, and is perhaps the most important mineral deficiency in ruminants after phosphorus (MORAES et al. 1999; VASQUEZ et al., 2001; RADOSTITS et al., 2007).

Among domestic species, sheep are undoubtedly the most predisposed to developing both deficiency and intoxication. These conditions are linked to marked differences in copper metabolism in certain breeds of sheep, because while some have a lower capacity to retain copper in their organic stores, others accumulate too much (SUTTLE, 2010; FERREIRA, ANTONELLI and ORTOLANI, 2008). It is also recognized that young growing sheep are much more susceptible to developing copper poisoning, as they can absorb dietary copper two to three times more efficiently than adults (SUTTLE, 2010).

Solaiman et al. (2006) in an experiment with goats, showed that for goats several factors, such as the initial copper status of the animals, the amount of copper and the concentration of its antagonists (Fe, S and Mo) in the basal diet, can affect the animals' responses to copper supplementation.

1.2 MINERAL SOURCES FOR RUMINANTS

The amount of minerals in fodder is quite variable, as it depends on the genus, species and variety of the plant, other factors such as the time of year, local climatic conditions, the amount of mineral in the soil and the type of soil and its conditions affect the absorption of minerals by the plant. The availability of elements in forage plants is largely affected by the presence of phytic and oxalic acid, normally found in cell walls formed by cellulose (HERRICK, 1993). All the minerals acquired by ruminants come entirely from the food ingested, since ruminants do not synthesize minerals (MENDONÇA JÛNIOR, 2011).

Whether accidentally, or due to a mineral deficiency, ruminants can also ingest minerals through the soil, a depraved appetite that characterizes allotrophagy and osteophagy, inducing the ingestion of materials foreign to their normal diet. Accidental soil ingestion can reach up to 20% of dry matter and is favored by poor drainage and weak soil structure, high stocking densities or during drought periods when pasture growth is excessively low. Soil ingestion can also lead to a copper deficiency due to the high consumption of Mo, Zn and other antagonists of this element present in the soil (McDOWELL, 1999).

The response to supplementation also depends on the mineral sources used in the process (CHAGAS et al., 2007).

Water is not considered a source of minerals, but it contains all the essential elements. Brackish water considerably reduces the consumption of mineral supplements due to its high sodium concentrations, leading to a consequent mineral deficiency in supplemented animals. High concentrations of sulphur observed in the water of deep aquifers obviously promote copper deficiency (MENDONÇA JÛNIOR, 2011).

1.3 COPPER METABOLISM AND STATUS IN RUMINANTS

The copper available in food is absorbed mainly in the small intestine, where soluble copper binds to certain amino acids that act as carriers of this element into the body. After entering the body, this mineral binds to albumin and is taken to the liver, the main storage site. From the liver, copper can have three destinations: it can be part of the hepatic stock within the hepatocytes; it can remain in the temporary stock bound to ceruloplasmin; or it can be excreted mainly through bile secretion (HOWELL and GOONERATNE, 1987).

According to Mills (1987), when the animal's consumption of copper falls short of its physiological need, its concentration and the activity of ceruloplasmin in the plasma are not reduced until the liver has a reserve of 40 mg/kg.

Well-conducted studies have shown that the availability of dietary copper can be drastically reduced in rations with high levels of molybdenum, sulphur and iron (VASQUEZ et al., 2001). Copper deficiency has been described in ruminants that receive these elements in high concentrations in the diet (MARQUES et al., 2003). On the other hand, a chemical compound known as tetrathiomolybdate, which has a high copper chelating power, has been used to treat copper intoxication in sheep (MACHADO, 1998; ORTOLANI, 2003; FERREIRA, ANTONELLI and ORTOLANI, 2008; SUTTLE, 2010).

The availability of dietary copper is also closely linked to the chemical form in which it is present in the food. The availability of the element in metallic form is reduced, although when it is associated with proteins or amino acids, absorption can sometimes be increased, and is very high in salt form (sulphate, carbonate, edetate). Surprisingly, in natura grasses have copper in metallic form, while the process of haying or ensiling the same grass causes part of this element to combine with proteins, facilitating absorption (ORTOLANI, 2003; SUTTLE, 2010).

Daily dietary copper requirements for sheep vary from 3 to 14 ppm, depending on the breed, and can triple during pregnancy and double during the lactation period (NRC, 2007). In most cases, copper deficiency can be primary, when the intake of this micromineral in the diet is low compared to the need for this element in the metabolic processes of the various classes of sheep. It can also be secondary when, despite adequate intake, its assimilation by the tissues is reduced by the presence of antagonistic elements in the diet, such as sulphur, iron and molybdenum. Goats can also be deficient in copper in regions with a certain deficiency of this mineral or too much of its antagonists in the soil and plants (SUTTLE 1986; GENGELBACH et al., 1994; RADOSTITS et al., 2007).

Copper deficiency in sheep and goats can cause: weakness and loss of waviness or depigmentation of the wool or black hair; congenital or contracted myelin alterations (enzootic ataxia) in which lambs and kids in the first weeks of life show incoordination of the hind limbs, which can result in paraplegia and death; osteoporosis; anemia; low immunity to infectious diseases and reduced growth (TOKARNIA et al., 1966; MAXIE, 2007; SUTTLE, 2010).

In Brazil, enzootic ataxia in sheep was first described in the state of Piaui, and more recently in Pernambuco, an outbreak was described in sheep and goats. In the majority of these animals, the symptoms were incoordination of the pelvic limbs, frequent falls and difficulty keeping in station, decreased sensory and motor response in determining the sensory reflex in the interdigital region of the hind limbs. In some cases, paralysis of the forelimbs occurred, which preceded the onset of permanent spasticity of all the limbs (TOKARNIA et al. 1966; SANTOS et al., 2006).

Histological examinations revealed faint edema and cerebral congestion in all the necropsied animals. Hematoxylin/Eosin (HE) staining of the spinal cord revealed axonal degeneration, gliosis, spheroids, a slight mononuclear infiltrate and perivascular cuffs. While Luxol Fast Blue staining revealed areas of dysmyelination in the ventral horn regions of the spinal cord, in the cervical and lumbar regions. Lesions in the cerebellum were detected in younger goats (axonal degeneration and vacuolization of the white matter) (SANTOS et al., 2006).

In a recent study on diseases of the central nervous system in goats and sheep in the semi-arid region, a frequency of 3.17% was found for cases of enzootic ataxia. Histological analysis showed Wallerian degeneration of the white matter of the medulla, particularly in the ventral funicles, as well as loss of myelin in the white matter in the medulla sections. Serum copper levels (1.61 - 1.29 µmol/L) were well below normal for the goat species (GUEDES et al., 2007).

Although the best known nutritional cause of adverse effects on reproduction is energy supplementation, deficiency or excess of other specific nutrients, particularly vitamins (Vitamin A and Vitamin E) and minerals (selenium, phosphorus, manganese, cobalt, iron, copper, fluorine and iodine), have been shown to affect fertility (DAYRELL, 1991).

Kegley and Spears (1994) reported that copper is an indispensable element for animal growth and development and for preventing a large number of clinical and pathological disorders that affect various species, such as: infertility, anemia, alterations, enzootic or neonatal ataxia, heart failure, depigmentation and defective keratinization of hair and wool, and diarrhea.

Ashmead (1993) reports that cows fed on copper-deficient pasture had low fertility. These females had depressed or delayed oestrus. In some cases where there was only one pregnancy, the dam interrupted the pregnancy by expelling a small dead fetus.

According to Riet-Correa et al. (2006), hypocuprosis occurs mainly in grazing animals, due to the low availability of this element in pastures, reducing the amount that can be absorbed by the body even with an adequate concentration of copper in the forage. Sandy soils, poor in organic matter and heavily weathered, such as areas on sea or river coasts, are likely to result in copper-deficient pastures.

In order to control or prevent copper deficiency in sheep and goats, it is necessary to supplement the herd with this element orally or parenterally in regions where there is evidence of hypocuprosis, or where there is a clear loss of productivity due to copper deficiency (RIET-CORREA et al., 2006). This supplementation can be carried out by including 0.25 to 0.5% copper sulphate in the mineral salt, or directly with mineral salt suitable for sheep. Providing sheep with mineral salt specifically for cattle can cause copper poisoning (RIET-CORREA et al., 2006).

1.4 COPPER DEFICIENCY SITUATION IN BRAZIL AND THE NORTHEAST

In Brazil, there have been several studies on mineral deficiencies in cattle, as well as the most efficient and economical forms of supplementation (MCDOWELL, 1999; TOKARNIA et al., 2000). However, knowledge about mineral deficiencies in sheep and goats is limited, especially in the semi-arid region. In this region, so-called "complete" mineral mixtures are recommended all year round, indiscriminately, for both grazing and confined or semi-confined animals.

They are often supplemented with minerals that are not necessary and even act as antagonists for other elements, for example: molybdenum which antagonizes copper; iron which antagonizes phosphorus and copper; and sulphur which antagonizes copper and selenium. When iron, molybdenum or sulphur are added to the mixtures, copper requirements increase (SOUSA, 1981; MCDOWELL, 1999; TOKARNIA et al., 1999).

Several studies have been carried out in Brazil on copper levels in pastures and copper depletion in the liver and/or serum of ruminants. There are studies in Amapà (TOKARNIA et al., 1971), Amazonas (BARROS et al., 1981; MORAES et al., 1999), Cearà (TOKARNIA et al., 1968), Goiàs (LOPES et al., 1980), Maranhao (TOKARNIA et al., 1960, 1968; MORAES et al., 1999), Mato Grosso and Mato Grosso do Sul (TOKARNIA et al., 1971; FERNANDES and SANTIAGO, 1972; SOUSA et al., 1980; BRUM et al., 1987; POTT et al., 1989; MORAES et al., 1999), Minas Gerais (MORAES et al., 1999), Parà (TOKARNIA et al., 1968, 1971), Pernambuco (SANTOS et al., 2006; MARQUES, 2010), Piaui (TOKARNIA et al., 1960, 1966, 1968, 1971), Rio de Janeiro (TOKARNIA et al., 1971; MORAES et al., 1999), Rio Grande do Sul (TRINDADE et al., 1990; BONDAN et al., 1991; RIET-CORREA et al., 1993; MORAES et al., 1999) Roraima (TOKARNIA et al., 1968; SOUSA et al., 1989), Santa Catarina (TOKARNIA et al., 1971), and Sao Paulo (LISBÔA et al., 1996).

According to Chagas (2007), deficiencies of both macronutrients and micronutrients have been found in most Brazilian pastures, for example: phosphorus (70%), zinc (95%), sodium (98%), iodine (95%) and, in the specific case of sheep, the element copper is at the limit of deficiency in 80% of the forages analyzed.

Few studies have been carried out in the state of Pernambuco on copper deficiency, and the only deficiencies diagnosed in goats and sheep in the semi-arid region were in grazing animals (RIET-CORREA, 2004; SANTOS et al., 2006). In sheep slaughtered in an abattoir in the state of Pernambuco, serum and liver copper levels were on average lower than the limits considered normal for the species, indicating the need to supplement this mineral for animals raised in the state (MARQUES, 2010).

Riet-Correa (2004) considers it important to characterize the mineral status in the semi-arid northeast, making it possible to know the aspects of its deficiency in relation to the productive and reproductive aspects of the goat and sheep contingent, which would make it possible to control these deficiencies more effectively in different breeding systems, particularly in the state of Pernambuco.

Soil and forage plant analyses are extremely important for regional mapping of mineral deficiencies, but they are difficult to interpret due to the great interaction between the elements involved, as well as being difficult to carry out (McDOWELL, 1992).

Most of the time, mineral determinations in animal biological material are sufficient for the diagnosis of deficiencies, with the results being interpreted more quickly and with less risk of error (SUTTLE, 2010). Around 40% to 70% of the copper absorbed is stored in the liver (CORAH and IVES, 1991), so analysis of liver samples is highly reliable in diagnosing copper deficiency (TOKARNIA et al., 1999). Seasonal environmental variations should also be taken into account when evaluating mineral profiles (CARDOSO, 1997).

By diagnosing which essential minerals are deficient, it is possible to establish control measures such as selective supplementation, which is often required for different sheep and goat farming systems. As the goat and sheep farming agribusiness in the Northeast is extremely important for the regional economy, it is important to study such an important indicator of this sector as mineral supplementation, especially copper and its main antagonists.

1.5 BIOCHEMICAL PROFILE

Although the nutritional requirements of goats and sheep are relatively well-established, there is still little information on the nutritional needs of small ruminants reared in the countryside. Most of the information available consists of extrapolations calculated from bovine data. However, due to the specific physiological characteristics of goats, more studies are needed (AGUILERA et al., 1990) and the establishment of reference values is essential (SKINNER, 2001). In addition, the measurement of certain biochemical elements, as well as the activity of various enzymes in the blood, can help with diagnosis, prognosis and monitoring the treatment of animals (MORAIS et al., 2000). However, in order to correctly interpret laboratory results, it is necessary to establish normal reference values for the different species, breeds, sexes and ages of animals raised in different regions of Brazil (BARONI et al., 2001).

In production animals, high blood urea values can indicate diets with low energy contents, just as low blood urea levels can indicate diets with low crude protein values (GONZALEZ et al., 2000).

The liver is of fundamental importance to ruminants, as more than 90% of the glucose they use is obtained via hepatic gluconeogenesis, since almost every source of glucose ingested in the diet is fermented and used by rumen bacteria. The liver is also a storage organ for various microminerals, and in the event of liver damage, these stocks are compromised, which can lead to deficiency in the animal. Hepatic insufficiency can also lead to lower clearance of ammonia from protein metabolism, which increases the risk of developing urea/ammonia poisoning. In this way, determining the activity of liver enzymes as a way of monitoring the activity of the liver is fundamental for the clinical practice of ruminants. However, it is necessary to establish normal reference values.

OBJECTIVES

1.6 GENERAL

The aim of this project was to study the essential microminerals (copper, iron, molybdenum and zinc) in the blood and liver of sheep and goats raised in the Petrolina micro-region in the state of Pernambuco.

1.7 SPECiFIC

To find out the levels of copper and its main antagonists (iron, molybdenum and zinc) in the blood and liver of sheep and goats raised in the Petrolina micro-region in the state of Pernambuco, taking into account the following factors: seasonality, location, species and sex;

Check whether copper deficiency occurs in this micro-region of the state of Pernambuco and whether its status is directly related to the action of elements considered to be antagonists.

Establish reference values for serum aspartate amino transferase and gamma glutamyl transferase activities.

MATERIALS AND METHODS

5.1 SAMPLE PLAN AND SAMPLE CHARACTERISTICS

The blood and liver samples were obtained from animals sent to the Petrolina Municipal Abattoir, located in the Petrolina micro-region in the Sao Francisco region of the state of Pernambuco. In order to establish the relationship between the origin of the animals and the data obtained, the division of the state into regions was used, as established by the Pernambuco State Agricultural Defense and Inspection Agency.

Before the animals were slaughtered, they were classified according to species, sex and municipality of origin. This information was used as a criterion for including the animals to be slaughtered as a sample in this experiment, as only adult, healthy animals from the municipalities of the Petrolina micro-region (Afrânio, Cabrobó, Dormentes, Lagoa Grande, Orocó, Petrolina, Santa Maria da Boa Vista and Terra Nova) would be considered.

During the sampling period, only animals from properties located in the municipalities of Petrolina, Dormentes and Santa Maria da Boa Vista were sent for slaughter at the Petrolina Municipal Abattoir, the place determined for obtaining samples. Thus, only these three municipalities were part of our sampling, as shown in Figure 1.

Figure 1 - Location of the municipalities in the Petrolina micro-region where the animals to be used in this experiment come from.

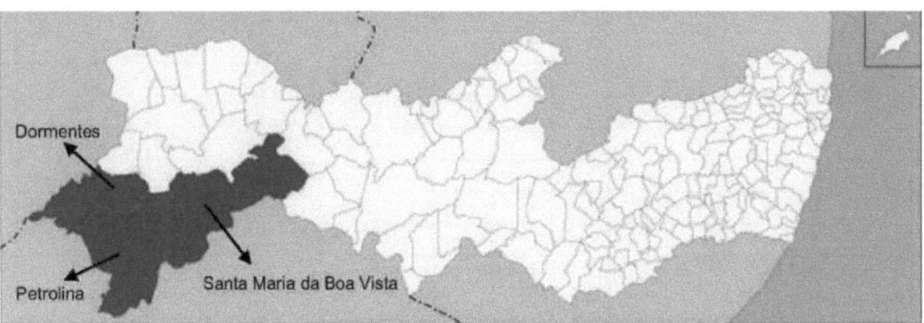

Fonte: http://pt.wikipedia.org/wiki/Ficheiro:Micro_Petrolina.png

Eighty animals of each species were selected at random, 20 males and 20 females during the rainy season and 20 males and 20 females during the dry season, giving a total of 160 animals at the end of the experiment.

The farms of origin of the animals selected for the experiment were visited to determine their coordinates (latitudeZlongitude) and consequently their location on a map of the region. During the visits, questionnaires were asked about the nutritional management used on each property in order to assess the influence of the areas and/or farming systems on the animals' mineral profile.

1.8 SAMPLE COLLECTION PERIOD

Samples were taken in two different periods (dry and rainy), considering the final third of each period. The purpose of this design was to characterize samples obtained during the period when nutrients are highly available to the animals (rainy) and during the period when the animal needs to mobilize reserves due to the lack of food (dry).

In order to define the dry and rainy periods in the Petrolina micro-region, we used data records of maximum and minimum temperatures and rainfall from the Meteorology Laboratory of Pernambuco (LAMEPE-ITEP), defined by the historical average for the region. In this way, it is possible to characterize the wettest months as being between November of one year and April of the following year, and the driest period as being between May and October of the same year.

Based on this data and considering only the final third of these periods, the collection months for the rainy season (PC) were defined as March and April, and for the dry season (PS) as September and October, as shown in Table 1 below.

Table 1 - Historical average rainfall (mm) for the months of the year for the municipalities in the Petrolina micro-region.

PCPS

Locations	JAN	FEB	MAR	APR	MAY	JUN	JUL	AUG	SET	OUT	NOV	TEN	ANNUAL
Afranio	72	87	143	80	13	7	2	2	7	23	52	85	**573**
Afrânio (Arizona)	62	77	103	67	12	5	1	1	3	14	50	58	**453**
Cabrobó	63	85	112	66	22	14	9	3	4	11	38	59	**486**
Dormant	109	86	123	97	33	7	3	2	8	15	59	68	**610**
Orocó	91	68	122	87	24	7	6	3	0	9	21	40	**478**
Petrolina	63	80	102	50	8	4	3	2	3	11	46	64	**436**
Petrolina (Rajada)	62	79	115	101	14	4	7	1	2	16	51	67	**519**
Santa Maria da Boa Vista	70	86	108	60	19	9	3	2	2	15	34	53	**461**
Terra Nova	90	139	158	120	39	16	14	4	5	19	36	75	**715**

Source: LAMEPE-ITEP (2011)

At the slaughterhouse, the animals were randomly selected by the person responsible for slaughtering them, respecting the inclusion criteria (species, sex and municipality of origin of the animal) (Figure 2).

Figure 2 - Animals to be slaughtered at the municipal slaughterhouse used in sampling

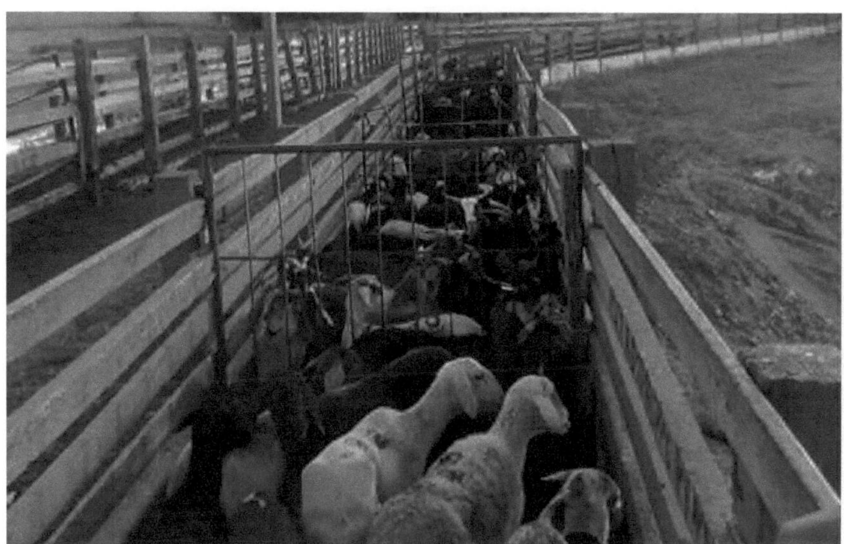

Source: Personal archive

5.3 COLLECTION OF BIOLOGICAL MATERIALS

Blood samples were collected by jugular venipuncture in siliconized vacuum collection tubes (Vacutainer®) without anticoagulants to obtain serum (Figure 3). After centrifugation for 15 minutes at 500 G, aliquots of serum were packed in quadruplicate in eppendorf tubes (2 ml) and stored at -20° C for mineral analysis and enzymatic activities.

The liver samples were obtained by cutting the organ into approximately 50 grams. The fragments were washed with sterile physiological solution, placed on filter paper to remove excess blood and water and placed in sterile universal collectors, duly identified, and stored in a freezer at -20° C.

Figure 3 - Blood collection before slaughter

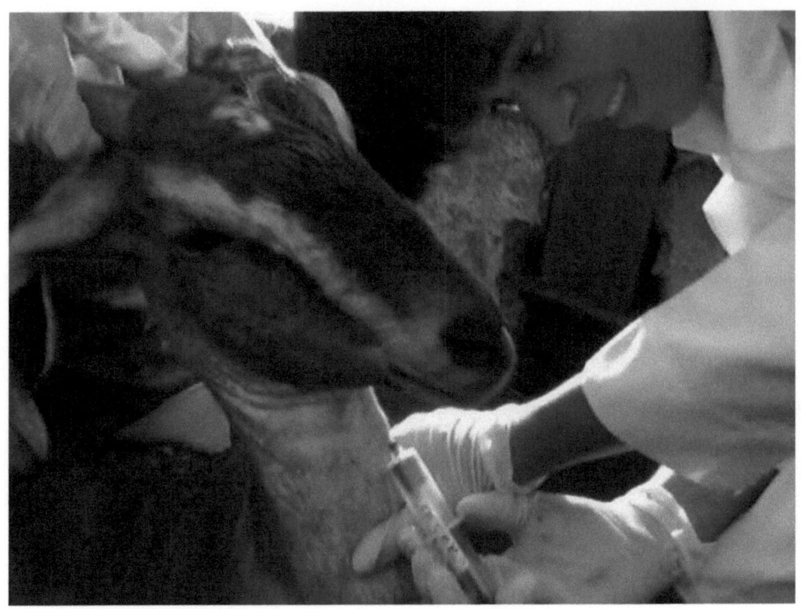

Source: Personal archive

5.4 LABORATORY ANALYSIS

Serum gamma glutamyltransferase (GGT), aspartate aminotransferase (AST), ceruloplasmin and copper, zinc, iron and molybdenum levels were determined. The biochemical analyses were processed using a Doles® model D-250 semi-automatic digital biochemical analyzer and a Celm® model E-225D digital spectrophotometer.

GGT activity was determined using a kinetic method, using the commercial Doles kit® .

AST activity was determined using a kinetic method, using the commercial Doles kit® .

Ceruloplasmin activity was determined using a colorimetric method according to Schosinsky et al. (1974) and adapted by López-Alonso et al. (2006). A buffer solution based on glacial acetic acid and sodium acetate, adjusted to a pH of 5.0, was prepared, as well as a substrate solution based on ortho-dianisidine and 50% sulfuric acid (9 mol/L). 750 μL of buffer solution was pipetted into two test tubes and 50 μL of serum was added to each, and they were incubated at 30° C for 5 minutes. After 5 minutes, 250 μL of the ortho-dianisidine-based substrate solution was added to each tube. The samples were incubated again at 30° C. After 5 minutes of incubation for one of the tubes and 15 minutes for the other tube, the absorbance is read at 580 nm on a spectrophotometer. From the values obtained, the following formula is applied to obtain the cerulopasmin activity value: (A15 - A5) x 6.25 x

100 IU/L.

To determine the minerals in the serum, they were diluted six to twenty times with Milli-Q water. To determine the concentrations of mineral elements in the liver, the samples were digested until a solution was obtained that retained the minerals of the initial sample and was completely liquid, without the presence of solid particles that could obstruct the spectrometer's suction capillaries and thus prevent the samples from being read, according to the recommendations of Tebaldi et al. (2000).

We therefore decided to carry out nitric-perchloric digestion in an open system. After thawing each organic sample at room temperature, it was subdivided into small pieces, placed in watch glasses, properly decontaminated and identified, and taken to an oven at 102°C for 24 hours. After drying, the samples were allowed to cool and then between 0.2 and 0.4 g of the dry sample was weighed using a high-precision balance. This sub-aliquot was transferred to 150 x 21 mm glass tubes, where 5 mL of a solution of nitric and perchloric acids were added in a ratio of 4:1, both P.A. acids.

The tubes containing the samples and the acid solution were left in a ventilated hood for 12 hours (*overnight*), after which the digestion process began. To do this, the tubes were placed in a digester block, which was operated at an initial temperature of 70° C for two hours, so that if there were any solid tissue particles left, they would be promptly solubilized. After this period, the temperature was increased to 150° C and kept there until digestion was complete, which was when all the acid had evaporated and all that remained was the mineral matter at the bottom of the tube, which should always be white in color. When, after the acid has evaporated, there is a dark color in the tube, the process should be repeated, as there is still organic matter to be digested.

After digestion, 20 mL of a 0.1 N hydrochloric acid solution was added to each tube. The solution was then homogenized vigorously and then placed in two 15 mL falcon tubes® . 10 mL of the solution was placed in each tube, then two equal aliquots of the same samples were read, one being analyzed and the other being used as a counter test.

The concentrations of copper, molybdenum, iron and zinc were determined using optical plasma emission spectrometry (ICP). Each time 20 samples were analyzed, an internal laboratory quality control was carried out (MILES *et al.*, 2001).

5.5 STATISTICAL ANALYSIS

Statistical analyses were processed using a computerized statistical program (MINITAB RELEASE 13, 2000).

The data obtained was first analyzed for its normal distribution using the Kolmogorov-Smirnov test (SIEGEL, 1975).

Depending on how far apart the data were, they were evaluated using parametric or non-parametric statistical tests. In the first case, the data was initially evaluated using the F test (analysis of variance), and when significant, the means were compared using the Duncan test (SAMPAIO, 1998). In the case of non-parametric data, they were analyzed using the Mann-Whitney test (SIEGEL, 1975). Differences where the "p" value was equal to or less than 0.05 ($p \leq 0.05$) were considered significant.

The Chi-Square test (MASSAD et al., 2004) was used to analyze the contingency table relating to the frequency of molybdenum levels.

To study the relationship between two variables, correlation coefficients were calculated (SNEDCOR and COCKRAN, 1967) and regression equations were obtained. It was established that there was a high intensity correlation between the variables when $r \geq 0.60$; medium intensity when $0.30 < r < 0.60$; and low intensity when $r \leq 0.30$, also considering that the level of significance obtained in the correlations was equal to or less than 5% (LITTLE and HILLS, 1978).

5.6 ETHICAL ASPECTS

This study was carried out in accordance with the ethical principles of animal experimentation, and the research project was approved by the Ethics Committee for Human and Animal Studies of the Federal University of Vale do Sâo Francisco (CEEHA/UNIVASF), protocol number 26101071.

RESULTS

Samples were collected during the months of September and October 2011, representing the dry season (DW), and during the months of March and April 2012, representing the rainy season (CW). All the animals were healthy and in good body condition. The slaughter of small ruminants at the Petrolina Municipal Abattoir takes place at night and weekly visits were made to the abattoir during the sampling periods to obtain the samples. In the afternoon, the animals were randomly selected, identified with ear tags and blood was collected. In the evening, the slaughter of the animals previously identified with earrings was monitored in order to collect fragments of the liver and thus relate the blood to the liver obtained.

Only animals from the municipalities of Petrolina, Dormentes and Santa Maria da Boa Vista were slaughtered at the abattoir, so the representativeness of the micro-region only includes these municipalities. Tables 1 and 2 show the distribution of animals by origin, where it can be seen that during the dry season most of the animals slaughtered at the municipal abattoir come from the municipality of Petrolina itself, since the sampling was proportional to the batches arriving at the abattoir.

Table 1 - Distribution of sheep sampled according to municipality of origin.

	Dry period			Rainy season		
Municipality	Male	Female	Total	Male	Female	Total
Dormant	4	5	9	8	8	16
Petrolina	13	12	25	8	8	16
Santa Maria da Boa Vista	3	3	6	4	4	8
Total	20	20	40	20	20	40

Table 2 - Distribution of the goats sampled according to municipality of origin.

Municipality	Dry period			Rainy season		
	Male	Female	Total	Male	Female	Total
Dormant	5	3	8	8	8	16
Petrolina	10	12	22	8	8	16
Santa Maria da Boa Vista	5	5	10	4	4	8
Total	20	20	40	20	20	40

The properties of origin of the animals participating in this study were traced, with 13 properties in total, divided into four properties in the municipality of Petrolina, seven properties in the municipality of Dormentes, and two properties in the municipality of Santa Maria da Boa Vista, whose location coordinates were determined using a GPS device and shown in Figure 2.

Figure 2 - Location of the farms from which the animals participating in the sampling originated.

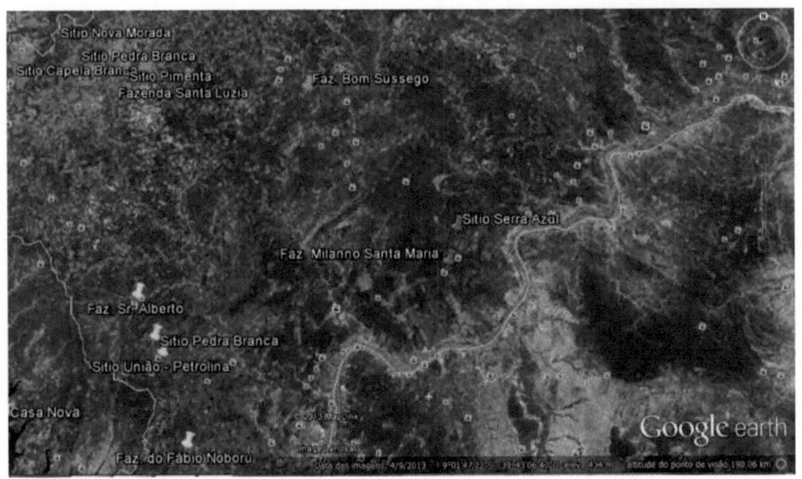

Source: Google Earth™

A questionnaire (Annex 1) was applied to each of the 13 farms in the municipalities of Petrolina, Dormentes and Santa Maria da Boa Vista, with the aim of obtaining information on the farming system applied on each of the farms.

Of the 13 properties analyzed, 61.5% kept their animals in a semi-extensive rearing system, released during the day and locked up at night, and the feed was based on native vegetation (caatinga). On these properties that raised animals in a semi-extensive system, 87.5% supplemented with commercial mineral salt, while 62.5% offered their own mineral salt for goats and/or sheep and 37.5% bought salt specifically for cattle and gave it freely to all the animals. The remaining 12.5% of these properties offered only pure white salt, which was placed freely in the trough inside the pens with free access to the animals.

The remaining 38.5% of farms used the extensive to ultra-extensive system, where the animals are raised loose in collective pastures or open areas, and only when they are sold are they collected and tied up for transport. None of these farms supplemented with mineral salt.

Of the 13 farms surveyed, 38.45% reported that some animals showed symptoms suggestive of copper deficiency, such as sudden death, malformation and incoordination of kids and lambs, pale mucous membranes, prostration, tremors and sudden death in young and adult animals. Of these properties, 40% provided mineral supplements, with one supplying mineral salt for cattle and the other only pure white salt.

The other 60% of farms that reported symptoms suggestive of copper deficiency did not offer any supplementation, as the animals were raised extensively. Symptoms on these farms were only detected at calving time or in outbreaks, and only the sick animals were separated and locked up for treatment.

Of the four properties located in the municipality of Petrolina, 25% reported that their animals had already shown symptoms suggestive of copper deficiency, even though they were supplied with mineral salt specifically for goats and sheep. In the municipality of Dormentes, of the seven properties visited, 42.85% reported the presence of symptoms suggesting the occurrence of copper deficiency in small ruminants. And in the municipality of Santa Maria da Boa Vista, 50% of the farms reported the presence of symptoms similar to copper deficiency among the animals. None of the 13 farms visited reported the occurrence of symptoms suggestive of cupric intoxication. A summary of the data obtained can be seen in Table 2.

Table 2 - Properties by municipality, farming system used and occurrence of symptoms suggestive of copper deficiency in small ruminants.

Municipality	Property	Breeding System	Occurrence of Symptoms
Petrolina	Mr. Alberto's farm	Semi Extensive	No
Petrolina	Fabio Noboru	Semi Extensive	No
Petrolina	Sitio Pedra Branca	Extensive	No
Petrolina	Sitio Uniao	Ultra Extensive	Yes
Dormant	Sitio Pimenta	Semi Extensive	No
Dormant	Sitio Nova Morada	Semi-extensive	No
Dormant	Sitio Capela Branca	Extensive	Yes
Dormant	Sitio Umburana	Semi-extensive	Yes
Dormant	Sitio Pedra Branca	Semi Extensive	No
Dormant	Santa Luzia Farm	Semi Extensive	No
Dormant	Bom Sucesso Farm	Extensive	Yes
Santa Maria da Boa Vista	Millano Farm	Semi Extensive	No
Santa Maria da Boa Vista	Sitio Serra Azul	Ultra Extensive	Yes

The serum copper values did not vary significantly when comparing the results obtained during the dry period with those obtained during the rainy period, in all the categories studied, but only when comparing the results obtained by the goats during the dry period did we see that the males had significantly higher values than the females, as shown in Table 3 and Graphs 1 and 2.

Table 3 - Mean values and standard deviations of serum copper content (μmol/L) in small ruminants from the Petrolina micro-region.

	Dry period	Rainy season

Male sheep	10,3±1,8	10,7±2,7
Female Sheep	10,7±2,0	9,8±1,5
Male goats	12,6±2,9^{A}	11,9±1,8
Female goats	10,2±2,4^{B}	11,3±2,2
Sheep Total	10,5±1,9	10,3±2,2
Goats Total	11,4±2,9	11,6±2,0

Note: Different capital letters in the columns indicate significant differences between the groups ($p < 0.05$).

Graph 1 - Average values of serum copper concentration (µmol/L) in small ruminants from the Petrolina micro-region, separated by sex and period.

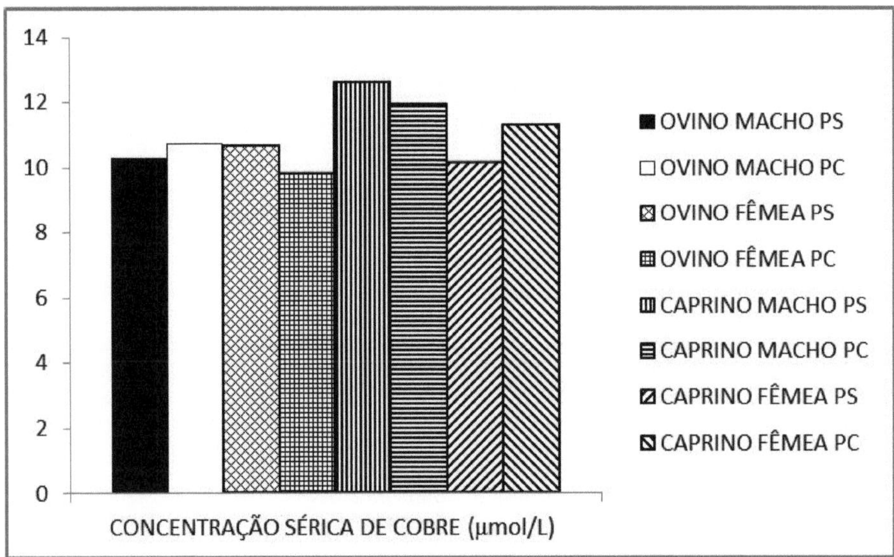

Graph 2 - Average values of serum copper concentration (µmol/L) in small ruminants from the Petrolina micro-region.

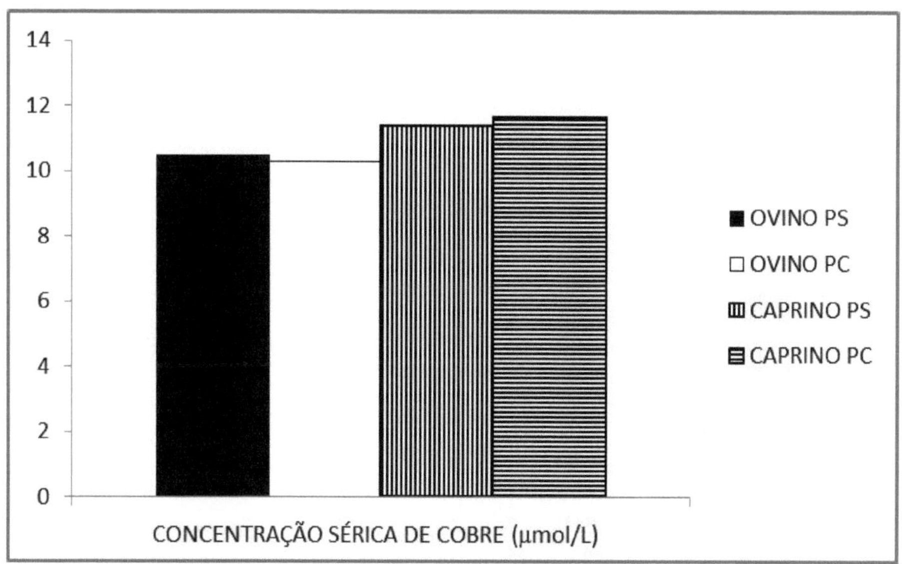

When we evaluated the serum zinc values, we found that there was no significant variation between the groups of sheep, either between the dry and rainy periods or between the sexes in the periods.

When we compared the results for the goats between the periods, while the males showed no significant difference, we found that the females showed significantly higher values in the rainy period than in the dry period. Likewise, when we compared the average values for all the goats, the rainy season showed significantly higher values than the dry season.

When comparing the values obtained by sheep and goats, it can be seen that sheep showed significantly higher average values than those obtained by goats in the dry period, while in the rainy period there was no significant difference between the species, as shown in Table 4 and Graphs 3 and 4.

Table 4 - Mean values and standard deviations of serum zinc content (µmol/L) in small ruminants from the Petrolina micro-region.

	Dry period	Rainy season
Male sheep	17,3±6,4	17,2±3,2
Female sheep	22,8±3,1	19,1±8,8
Male goats	15,8±3,7	21,0±9,3
Female goats	11,6±2,8^{b}	21,2±6,5^{a}
Sheep Total	20,2±5,6^{A}	18,1±6,5
Goats Total	13,7±3,9^{bB}	21,1±7,7^{a}

Note: Different lowercase letters in the rows indicate significant differences between the periods ($p < 0.05$). Different capital letters in the columns indicate significant differences between the groups ($p < 0.05$).

Graph 3 - Average values of serum zinc concentration (µmol/L) in small ruminants from the Petrolina micro-region, separated by sex and period.

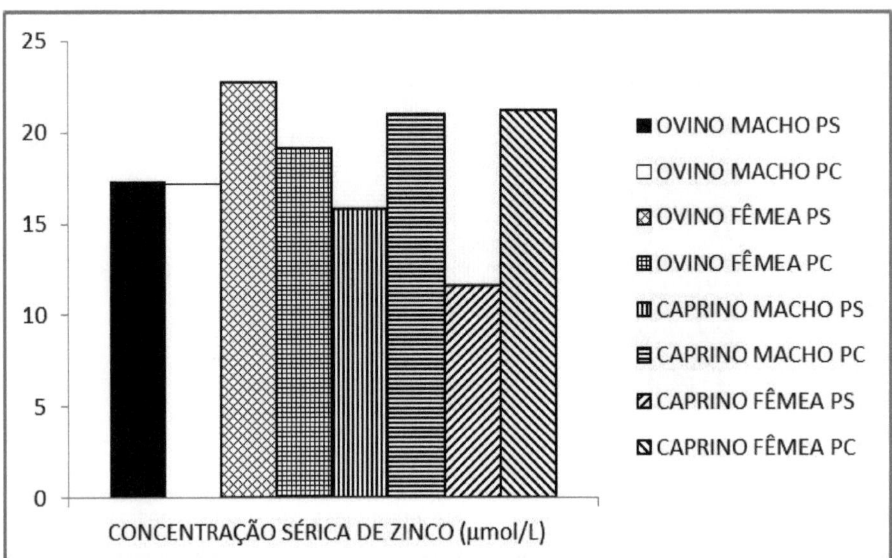

Graph 4 - Average values of serum zinc concentration (µmol/L) in small ruminants from the Petrolina micro-region.

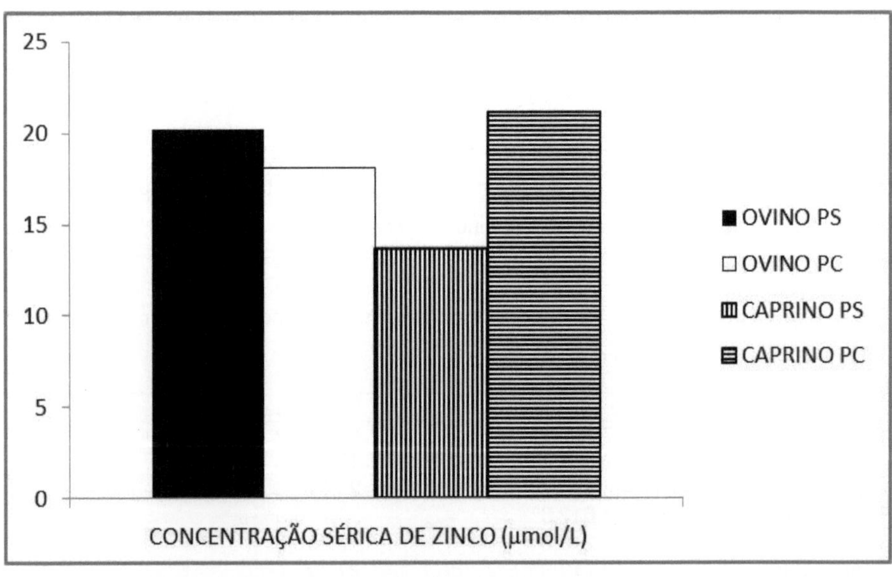

When analyzing the results for serum iron levels, it can be seen that sheep showed significantly higher average values in the dry period compared to the rainy period, both for males, females and sheep in general. There was no significant difference between male and female sheep in any period.

When we evaluated the results for goats, there was no significant difference between the dry and rainy periods for males, females and goats in general.

When comparing the average serum iron values obtained by sheep and goats, it can be seen that sheep showed significantly higher average values than goats in the dry period, while in the rainy period there was no significant difference between the species, as shown in Table 5 and Graphs 5 and 6.

Table 5 - Mean values and standard deviations of serum iron content (□mol/L) in small ruminants from the Petrolina micro-region.

	Dry period	Rainy season
Male sheep	74,0±25,2[a]	48,3±13,1[b]
Female Sheep	82,5±30,1[a]	54,3±21,9[b]
Male goats	51,5±20,2	43,6±12,1
Female goats	39,3±15,0	49,2±7,3
Sheep Total	78,5±27,8[aA]	51,2±18,0[b]
Goats Total	45,4±18,5[B]	46,4±10,3

Note: Different lowercase letters in the rows indicate significant differences between the periods ($p < 0.05$). Different capital letters in the columns indicate significant differences between the groups ($p < 0.05$).

Graph 5 - Average values of serum iron concentration (µmol/L) in small ruminants from the Petrolina micro-region, separated by sex and period.

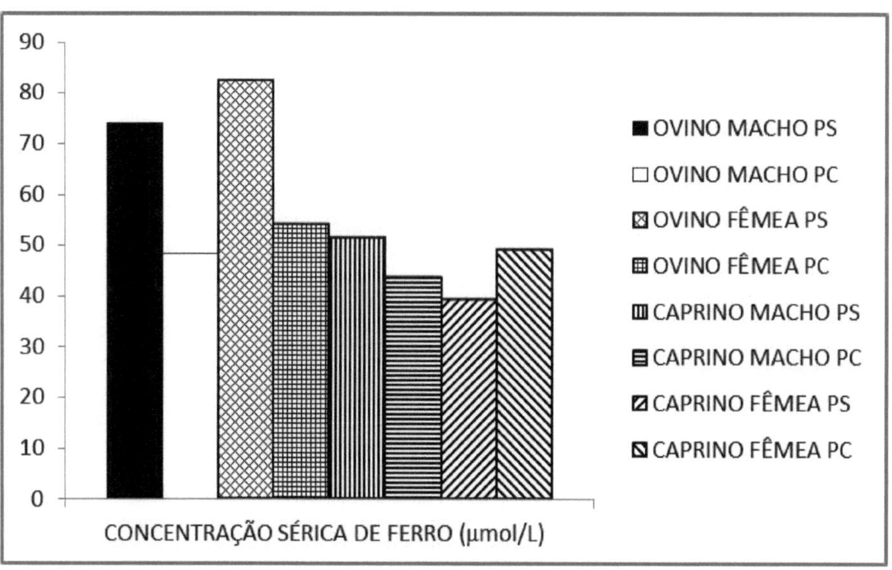

Graph 6 - Average values of serum iron concentration (µmol/L) in small ruminants from the Petrolina micro-region.

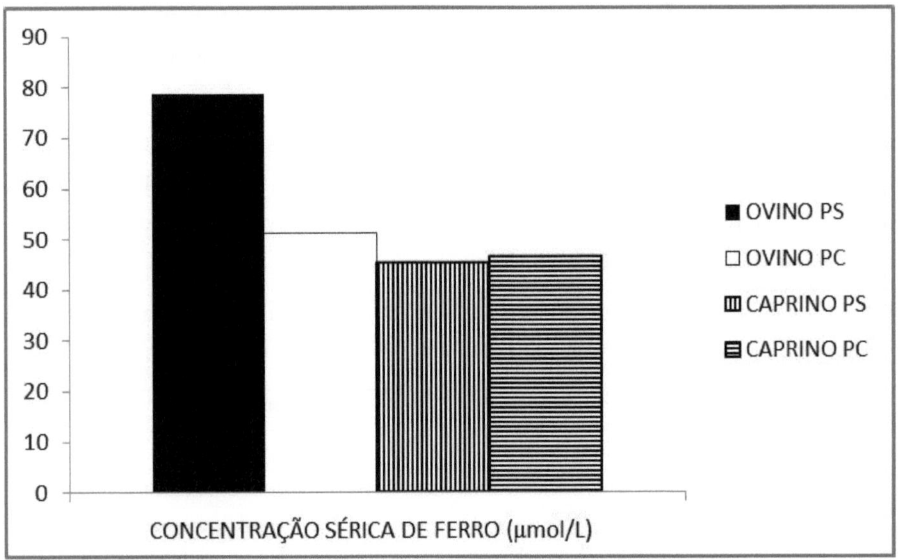

In a significant proportion of the samples, the serum molybdenum content was below the calibration and determination threshold of the optical plasma emission spectrometry apparatus used in this experiment, and so the statistical analysis for this variable was carried out in a differentiated way, using the Chi-Square test in order to compare the proportions of each category varying in sex, period and molybdenum content greater or less than 0.05 µmol/L, as shown in Table 6.

Table 6 - Frequency of animals with serum molybdenum levels above and below 0.05 µmol/L in small ruminants from the Petrolina micro-region.

	Dry period > 0.05< 0.05	Rainy season > 0.05< 0.05	*p-value*
Male sheep	137	614	0,0267
Female Sheep	020	812	0,0016
p-value	< 0,0001	0,5073	
Male goats	911	713	0,5186
Female goats	317	020	0,0717
p-value	0,0384	0,0036	
Sheep Total	1327	1426	0,8131
Goats Total	1228	733	0,1890
p-value	0,8094	0,0753	

Note: p-value in the row for the difference between periods. P-value in the column in the 1ª and 2ª sections for the difference between sexes, and in the 3ª section for the difference between species.

Thus, we found that there was a decrease in the frequency of male sheep with molybdenum content above 0.05 μmol/L in the rainy period compared to the dry period, while the opposite occurred with females. When we look at the influence of gender, we see that only in the

During the dry period, there was a significant difference, with males having a higher number of animals with molybdenum content above 0.05 μmol/L, while females had more animals with content below this value.

With regard to the goats, we found that there was no influence of the period on the number of animals in relation to the serum molybdenum content, but it was found that in both periods the number of male goats with a molybdenum content above 0.05 μmol/L was higher than that of female goats.

There was no significant difference in frequency between species, nor between periods when the sex factor was not taken into account.

We were able to comparatively analyze the averages of the samples in which the molybdenum levels were above 0.05 μmol/L (except for female sheep in the dry period and female goats in the rainy period), and there was no significant difference between male and female sheep in any of the periods, nor was there any difference between the periods. When we evaluated the results obtained by the goats, there were also no significant differences at any time. There were also no differences between the species in any of the periods, as shown in Table 7.

Table 7 - Mean values and standard deviation (μmol/L) of serum molybdenum in animals with a content above 0.05 μmol/L in small ruminants from the Petrolina micro-region.

	Dry period	Rainy season
Male sheep	0,16±0,10	0,20±0,08
Female sheep	-	0,12±0,06
Male goats	0,16±0,08	0,10±0,05
Female goats	0,20±0,04	-
Sheep Total	0,16±0,10	0,10±0,05
Goats Total	0,17±0,08	0,15±0,08

Note: There was no significant difference between the groups or between the periods.

The hepatic copper values did not vary significantly when comparing the results obtained during the dry period with those obtained during the rainy period, in all the categories studied, and there were no differences between the species in any of the periods, as shown in Table 8 and Graphs 7 and 8.

Table 8 - Mean values and standard deviations of hepatic copper content (ppm) in small ruminants from the Petrolina micro-region.

	Dry period	Rainy season
Male sheep	217±133	236±110
Female Sheep	245±173	295±206
Male goats	210±133	295±163
Female goats	211±114	266±147
Sheep Total	230±151	266±166
Goats Total	211±120	280±154

Note: There was no significant difference between the groups or between the periods.

Graph 7 - Average values of hepatic copper content (ppm) in small ruminants from the Petrolina micro-region, separated by sex and period.

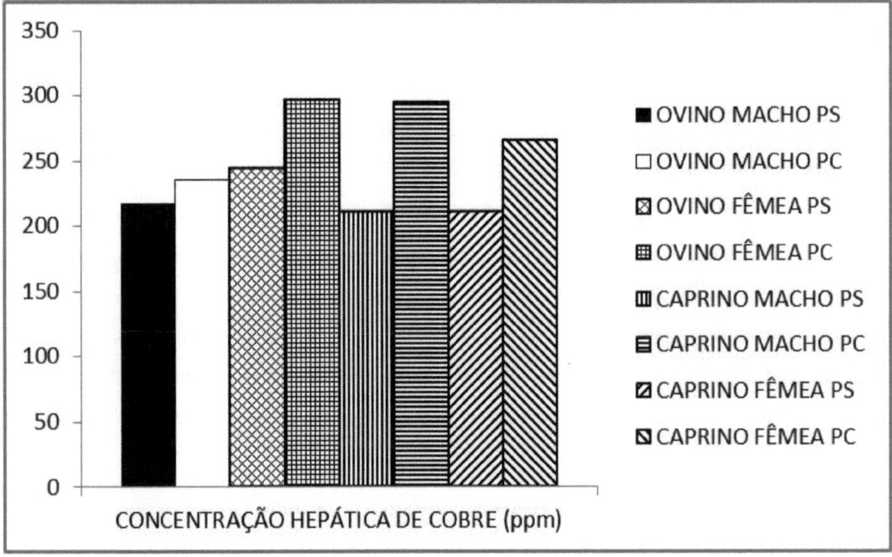

Graph 8 - Average values of hepatic copper content (ppm) in small ruminants from the Petrolina micro-region.

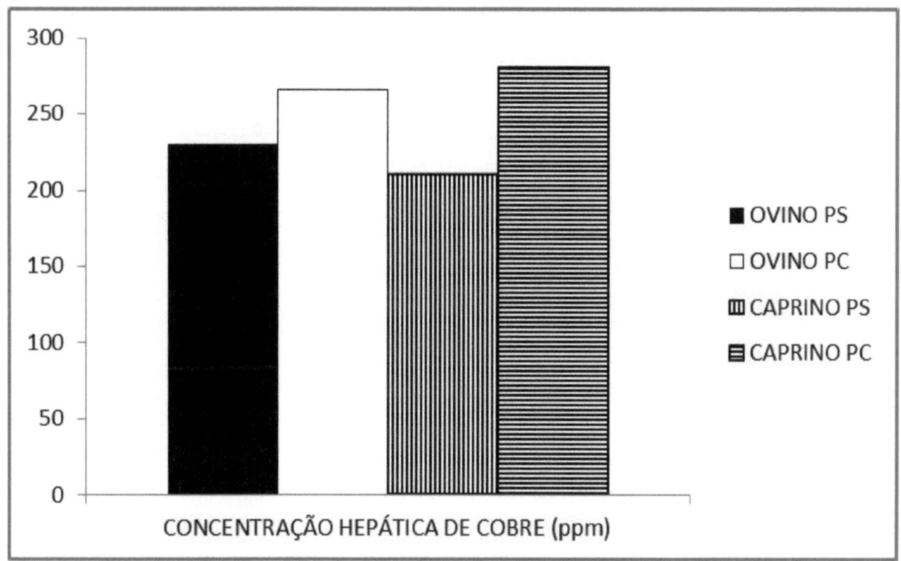

When we evaluated the hepatic values of zinc in sheep, we found that there was a significant variation only between males from the dry period and those from the rainy period, where the latter had higher average values. There was no significant difference between males and females.

When we compared the results for goats between the periods or between the sexes in each period, there were no significant differences, nor were there any differences between the species in any of the periods, as shown in Table 9 and Graphs 9 and 10.

Table 9 - Mean values and standard deviations of hepatic zinc content (ppm) in small ruminants from the Petrolina micro-region.

	Dry period	Rainy season
Male sheep	104±21[b]	133±50[a]
Female Sheep	111±19	110±20
Male goats	118±21	111±163
Female goats	107±22	109±18
Sheep Total	107±20	122±39
Goats Total	113±22	110±21

Note: Different lower-case letters in the lines indicate significant differences between the periods ($p < 0.05$).

Graph 9 - Average values of hepatic zinc content (ppm) in small ruminants from the Petrolina micro-region, separated by sex and period.

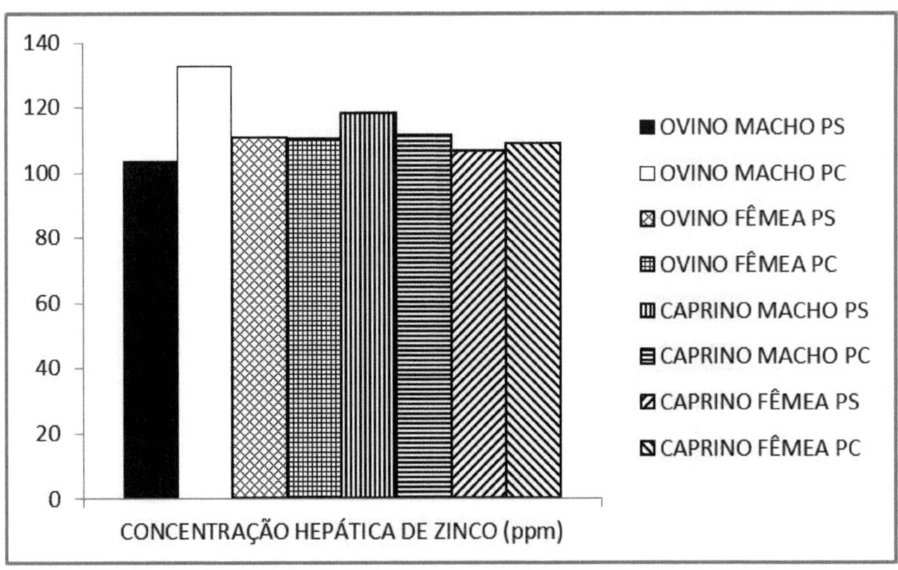

Graph 10 - Average values of hepatic zinc content (ppm) in small ruminants from the Petrolina micro-region.

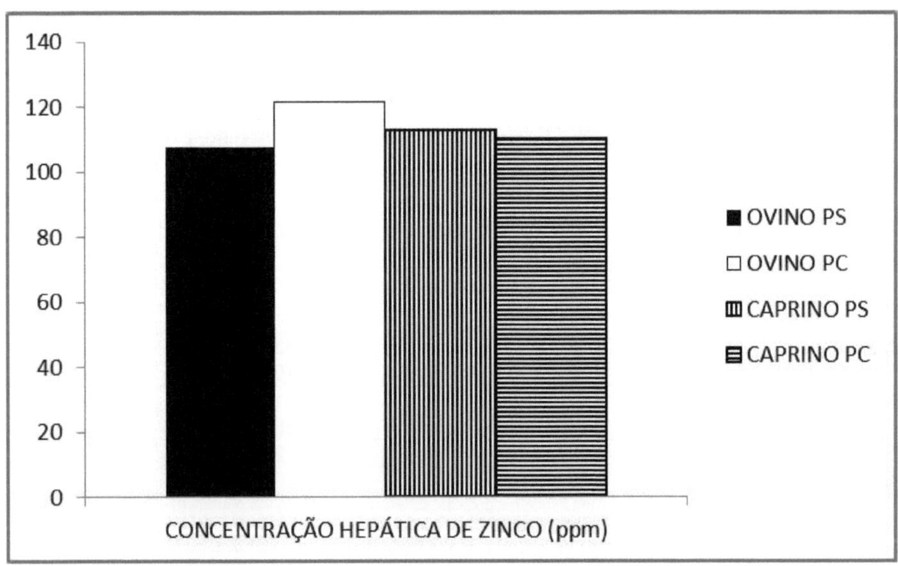

When evaluating hepatic iron levels, both sheep and goats showed no significant variation when comparing the average values obtained during the dry period with those obtained during the rainy period, in all the categories studied.

When comparing the species, sheep showed significantly higher mean hepatic iron values than goats in both the dry and rainy periods, as shown in Table 10 and Graphs 11 and 12.

Table 10 - Mean values and standard deviations of hepatic iron content (ppm) in small ruminants from the Petrolina micro-region.

	Dry period	Rainy season
Male sheep	267±113	225±101
Female Sheep	233±103	255±116
Male goats	136±53	145±64
Female goats	162±42	155±68
Sheep Total	250±108^{A}	240±108^{A}
Goats Total	149±49^{B}	150±66^{B}

Note: Different capital letters in the columns indicate significant differences between the groups ($p < 0.05$).

Graph 11 - Average values of hepatic iron content (ppm) in small ruminants from the Petrolina micro-region, separated by sex and period.

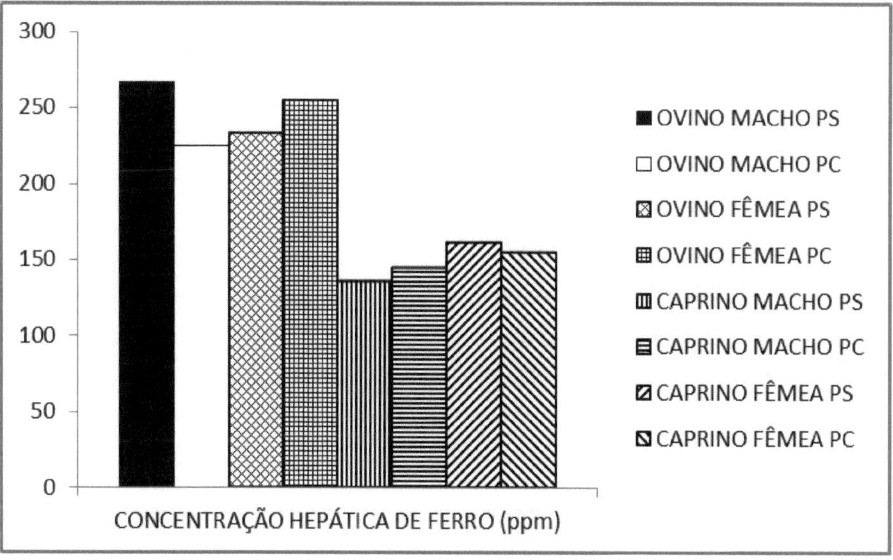

Graph 12 - Average values of hepatic iron content (ppm) in small ruminants from the Petrolina micro-region.

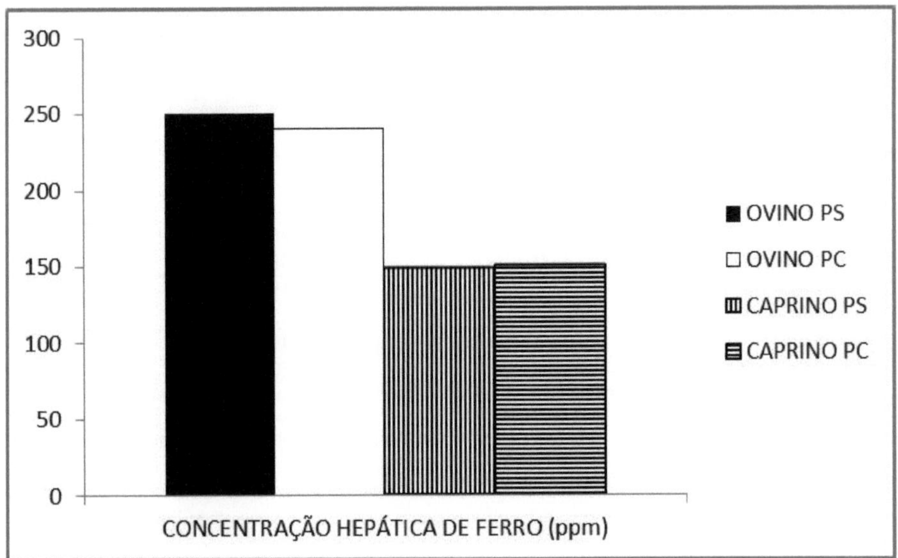

When evaluating the hepatic molybdenum levels in sheep, it can be seen that females showed significantly higher average values in the dry period compared to the rainy period, a fact that did not occur with males and females. When comparing the sexes within each period, there was no significant difference between male and female sheep, nor when comparing sheep in general between the dry and rainy periods.

When analyzing the results for goats, both males and females showed significantly higher average values in the dry period compared to the rainy period, with no significant difference between the sexes in either period. When comparing goats in general, the dry period showed significantly higher average values than the rainy period.

When comparing the average hepatic molybdenum values obtained by sheep and goats, it can be seen that the sheep showed significantly higher average values than those obtained by the goats during both the dry and rainy periods, as shown in Table 11 and Graphs 13 and 14.

Table 11 - Mean values and standard deviations of hepatic molybdenum content (ppm) in small ruminants from the Petrolina micro-region.

	Dry period	Rainy season
Male sheep	3,0±1,1	3,1±0,6
Female Sheep	3,3±1,3^{a}	2,4±0,8^{b}
Male goats	2,7±1,1^{a}	0,8±0,5^{b}
Female goats	2,4±0,9^{a}	0,9±0,8^{b}
Sheep Total	3,2±1,2^{A}	2,7±0,8^{A}

Goats Total	$2,5\pm1,0^{aB}$	$0,8\pm0,7^{bB}$

Note: Distinct lowercase letters in the rows indicate significant differences between the periods ($p < 0.05$). Distinct capital letters in the columns indicate significant differences between the groups ($p < 0.05$).

Graph 13 - Average values of hepatic molybdenum content (ppm) in small ruminants from the Petrolina micro-region, separated by sex and period.

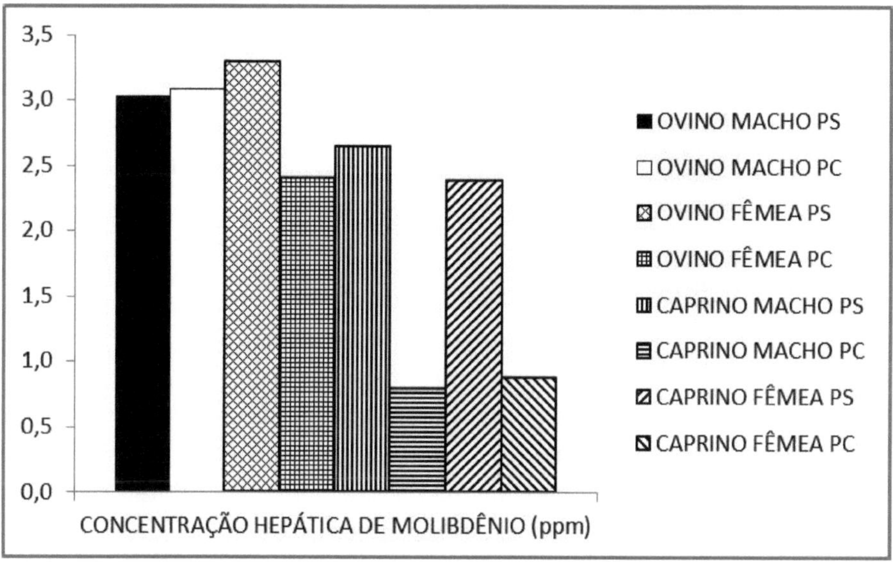

Graph 14 - Average values of hepatic molybdenum content (ppm) in small ruminants from the Petrolina micro-region.

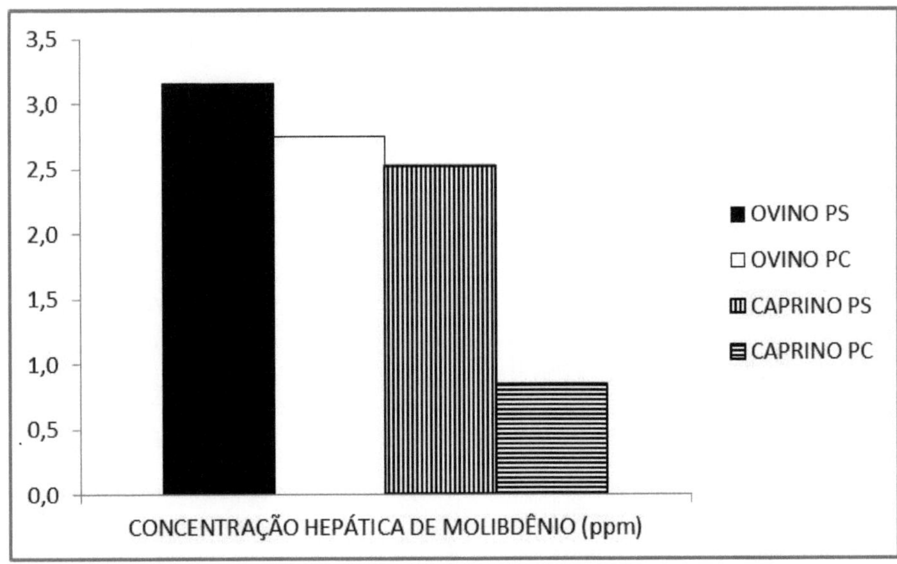

When analyzing the results for serum ceruloplasmin activity, it can be seen that both male and female sheep and goats showed significantly higher average values in the rainy season compared to the dry season. There was no significant difference between males and females of either species during the rainy or dry periods.

When comparing the average values obtained between the species, it was determined that goats had higher values than sheep in general during the rainy season, while during the dry season there was no significant difference.

Table 12 - Mean values and standard deviations of Ceruloplasmin serum activity (UI/L) in small ruminants from the Petrolina micro-region.

	Dry period	Rainy season
Male sheep	7,9±4,8[b]	22,2±15,8[a]
Female sheep	11,1±5,8[b]	19,6±6,8[a]
Male goats	10,3±6,5[b]	28,7±9,3[a]
Female goats	5,8±4,4[b]	28,9±11,6[a]
Sheep Total	9,5±5,5[b]	20,9±12,0[aB]
Goats Total	8,1±5,9[b]	28,8±10,4[aA]

Note: Distinct lower-case letters in the rows indicate significant differences between the periods ($p < 0.05$). Distinct capital letters in the columns indicate significant differences between the groups ($p < 0.05$).

Graph 15 - Average values of serum Ceruloplasmin activity (IU/L) in small ruminants from the Petrolina micro-region, separated by sex and period.

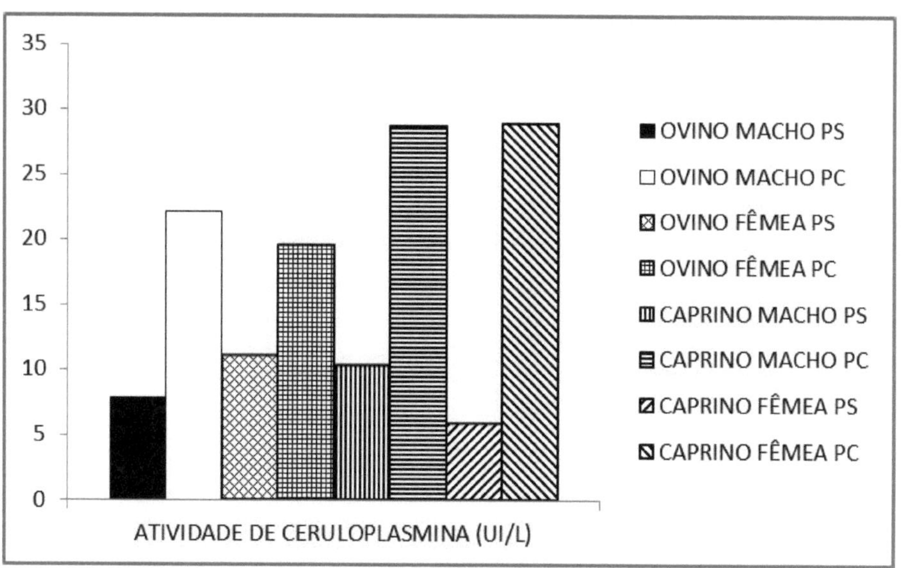

Graph 16 - Average values of Ceruloplasmin serum activity (IU/L) in small ruminants from the Petrolina micro-region.

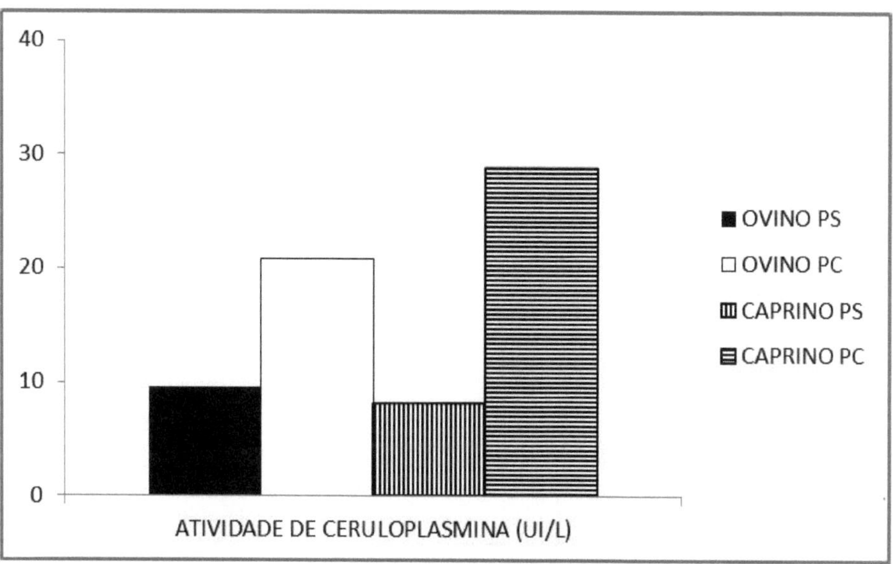

The results of serum GGT activity show that male sheep had higher average values in the rainy season than males in the dry season, as well as females in the rainy season. There was no significant difference between females in the different periods, or between males and females in the dry period.

When we evaluated the average values of this enzyme's activity in goats, we found that females showed a significant difference, with animals from the rainy season showing higher average values than those from the dry season.

The same significant pattern was observed in goats in general, where animals from the rainy period had higher GGT activity values than those from the dry period. Sheep in general, on the other hand, showed no significant difference between the periods, or when comparing sheep and goats in the two periods.

Table 13 - Mean values and standard deviations of serum GGT activity (IU/L) in small ruminants from the Petrolina micro-region.

	Dry period	Rainy season
Male sheep	$39,6 \pm 10,0^{b}$	$62,3 \pm 17,4^{aA}$
Female Sheep	$43,3 \pm 10,8$	$32,7 \pm 17,7^{B}$
Male goats	$37,1 \pm 15,8$	$47,9 \pm 9,4$
Female goats	$31,7 \pm 9,8^{b}$	$46,7 \pm 8,4^{a}$
Sheep Total	$41,4 \pm 10,5$	$46,7 \pm 22,9$
Goats Total	$34,4 \pm 13,3^{b}$	$47,3 \pm 8,9^{a}$

Note: Distinct lowercase letters in the rows indicate significant differences between the periods ($p < 0.05$). Distinct capital letters in the columns indicate significant differences between the groups ($p < 0.05$).

Graph 17 - Average values of serum GGT activity (IU/L) in small ruminants from the Petrolina micro-region, separated by sex and period.

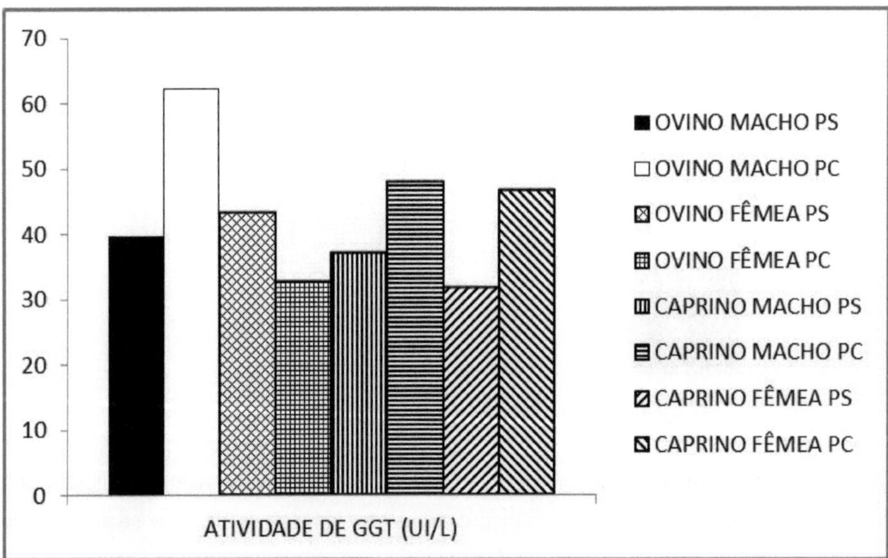

Graph 18 - Average values of serum GGT activity (IU/L) in small ruminants from the Petrolina micro-region.

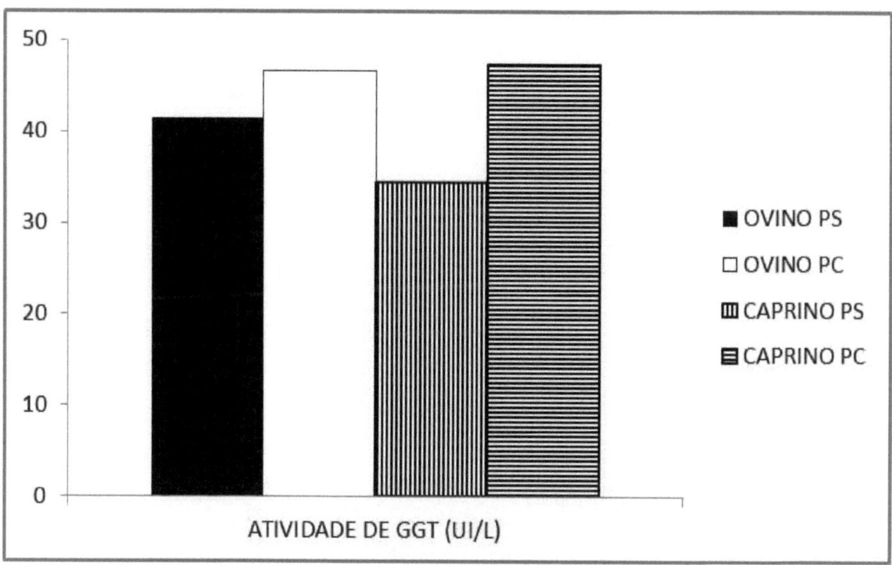

The results of serum AST activity in sheep show that females in the dry period had higher median values than females in the rainy period. Males in the rainy period had higher median AST activity values than females in the same period. There was no significant difference between males or sexes in the dry period.

When we evaluated the median values of this enzyme's activity in goats, we found that only males showed a significant difference, with animals from the rainy season showing higher median values than those from the dry season. There was no difference between females and there was no significant difference between males and females in either period.

When we evaluated the values obtained for sheep and goats by grouping males and females, we found that goats from the rainy season had higher median values than goats from the dry season, as well as higher values than sheep from the rainy season, as can be seen in Table 14 and Graphs 19 and 20.

Table 14 - Medians, P25 and P75 of serum AST activity (IU/L) in small ruminants from the Petrolina micro-region.

	Dry period	Rainy season
Male sheep	103,1 (85,4 - 131,3)	126.4 (103.8 - 172.0)^{A} 74.1
Female Sheep	108,4 (92,1 - 127,9) ^{a}	(42.5 - 93.5) ^{bB}
Male goats	73.5 (69.5 - 85.1)^{b} 105.1 (71.4 -116,7 (99,9 - 153,8) ^{a}	

Female goats	155.7)	136,0 (115,4 - 149,3)
Sheep Total	107,6 (87,2 - 130,7)	96.3 (72.6 - 144.3)^B 131.6
Goats Total	83,0 (69,2 - 135,9) ^{b}	(107.1 - 151.7) ^{aA}

Note: Distinct lowercase letters in the rows indicate significant differences between the periods ($p < 0.05$). Distinct capital letters in the columns indicate significant differences between the groups ($p < 0.05$).

Graph 19 - Medians of serum AST activity (IU/L) in small ruminants from the Petrolina micro-region, separated by sex and period.

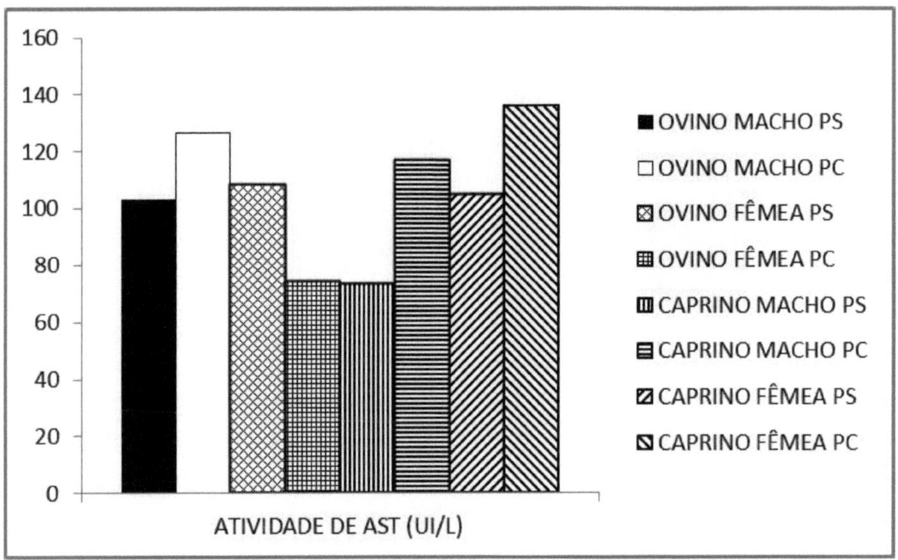

Graph 20 - Average values of serum AST activity (IU/L) in small ruminants from the Petrolina micro-region

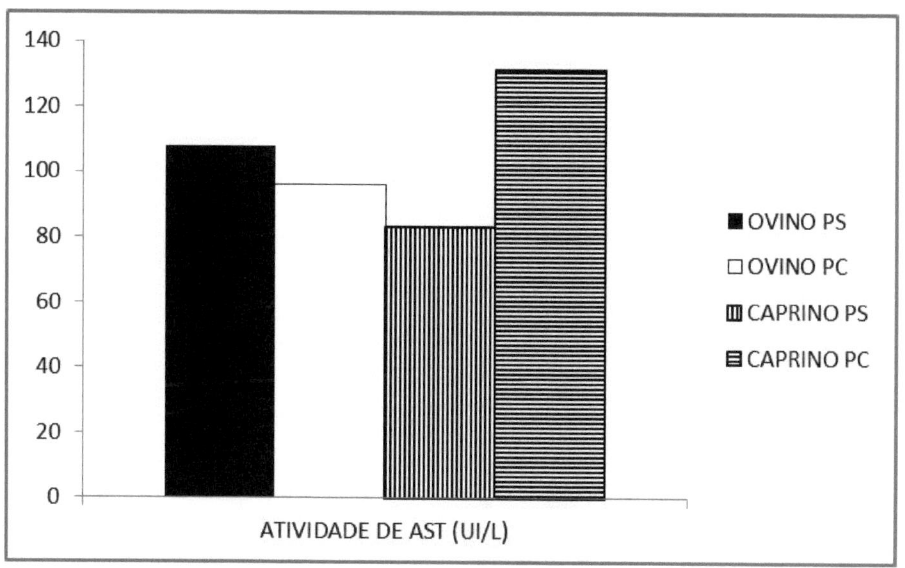

The analysis of the relationship between serum copper and liver copper showed a low positive relationship (r = 0.06), and is expressed by the equation:

y = 0.0012x + 10.658

Graph 21 - Ratio of serum copper (μmol/L) to liver copper (ppm) in small ruminants from the Petrolina micro-region.

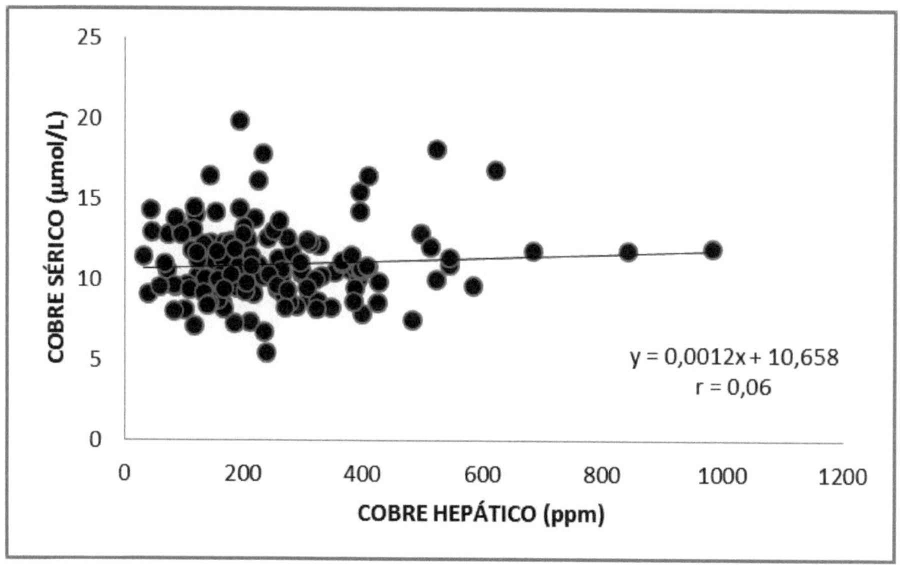

The analysis of the relationship between hepatic copper and hepatic zinc showed a low positive relationship (r = 0.22), and is expressed by the equation:

y = 1.2069x + 111.76

Graph 22 - Ratio of hepatic copper (ppm) to hepatic zinc (ppm) in small ruminants from the Petrolina micro-region.

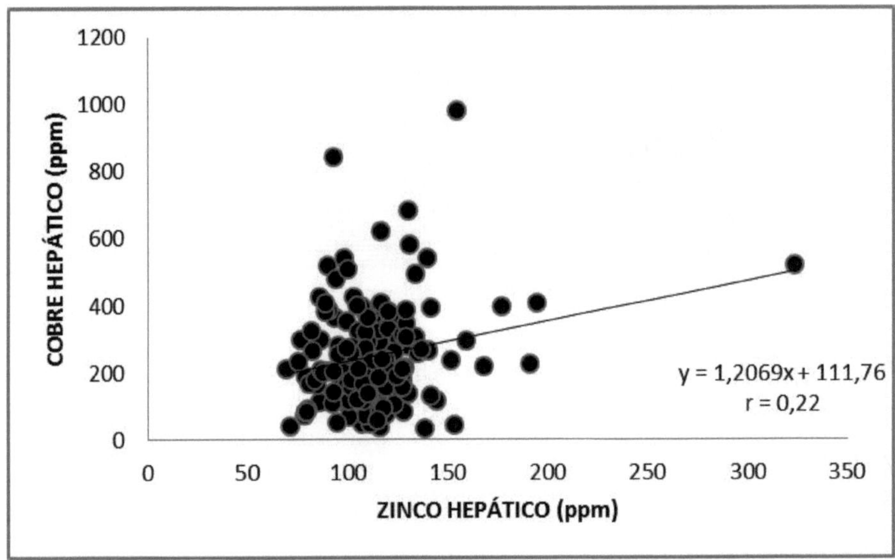

The analysis of the relationship between hepatic copper and hepatic iron showed a low positive relationship (r = 0.12), and is expressed by the equation:

y = 0.19x + 210.32

Graph 23 - Ratio of hepatic copper (ppm) to hepatic iron (ppm) in small ruminants from the Petrolina micro-region.

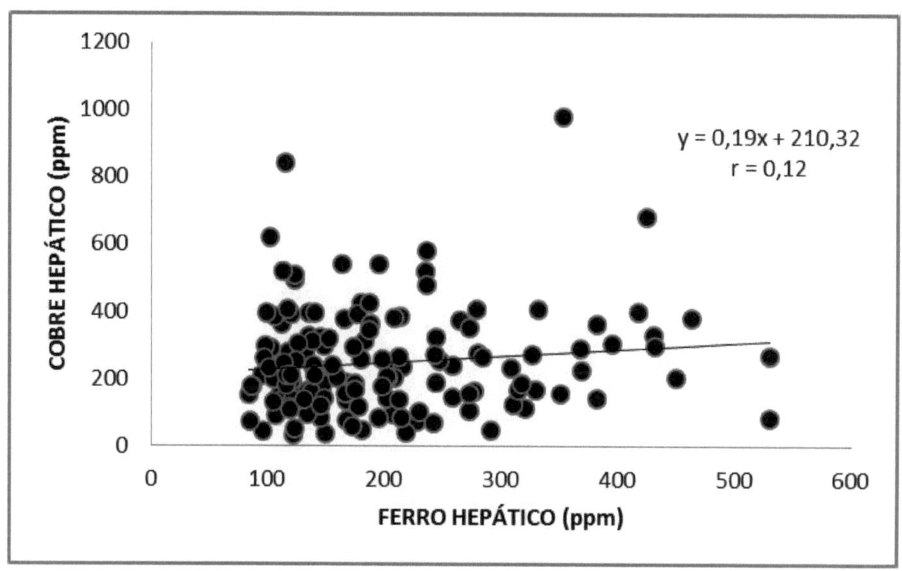

The analysis of the relationship between hepatic copper and hepatic molybdenum showed a low negative relationship (r = 0.14), and is expressed by the equation:

y = -17.002x + 279.6

Graph 24 - Ratio of hepatic copper (ppm) to hepatic molybdenum (ppm) in small ruminants from the Petrolina micro-region.

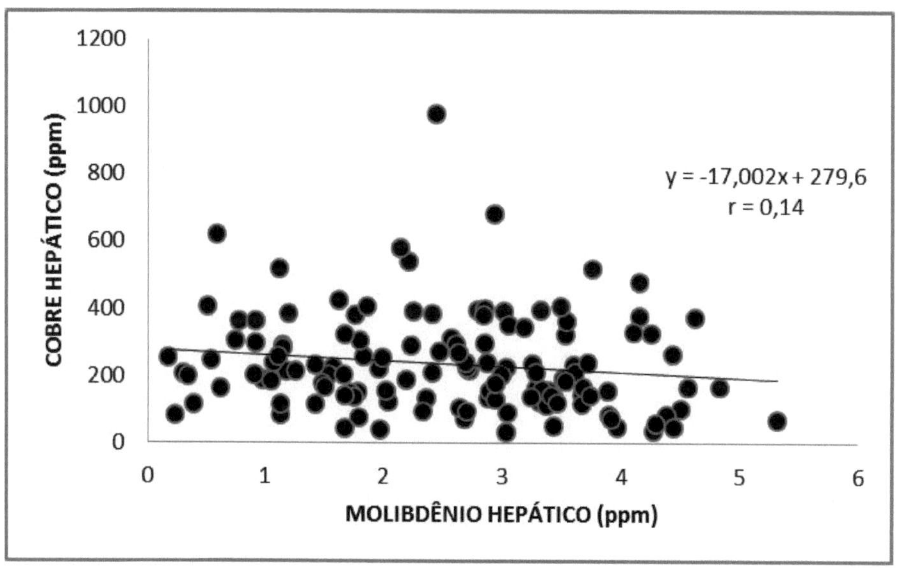

The analysis of the relationship between Ceruloplasmin activity and serum copper in sheep during the dry period showed a high positive relationship (r = 0.67), and is expressed by the equation:

y = 2.1024x - 12.291

Graph 25 - Relationship between ceruloplasmin activity (IU/L) and serum copper (μmol/L) in sheep during the dry season in the Petrolina micro-region.

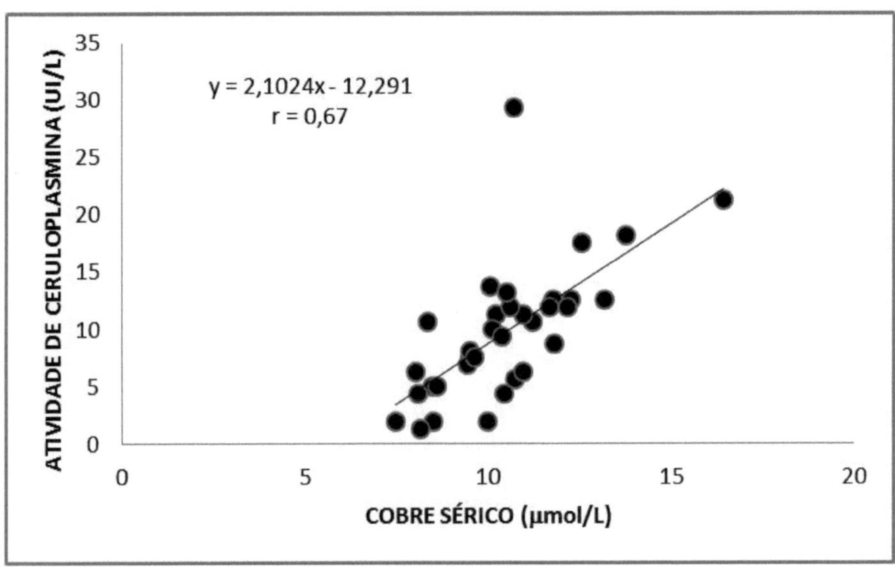

The analysis of the relationship between ceruloplasmin activity and serum copper in goats during the dry period showed a high positive relationship (r = 0.67), and is expressed by the equation:

y = 1.3978x - 7.2991

Graph 26 - Relationship between Ceruloplasmin activity (IU/L) and serum copper (μmol/L) in goats during the dry period.

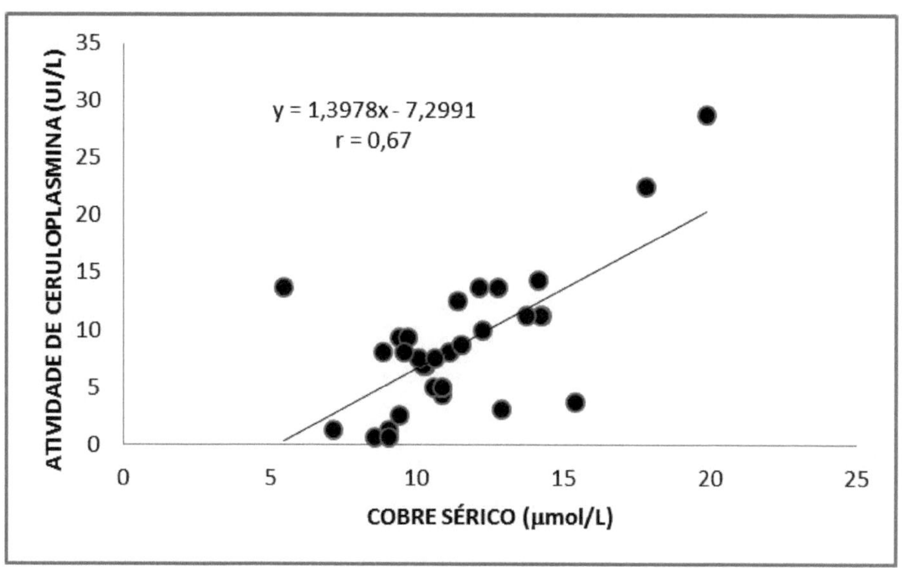

The analysis of the relationship between ceruloplasmin activity and serum copper in sheep during the rainy season showed a high positive relationship (r = 0.79), and is expressed by the equation:

y = 4.3195x - 23.441

Graph 27 - Relationship between ceruloplasmin activity (IU/L) and serum copper (µmol/L) in sheep during the rainy season.

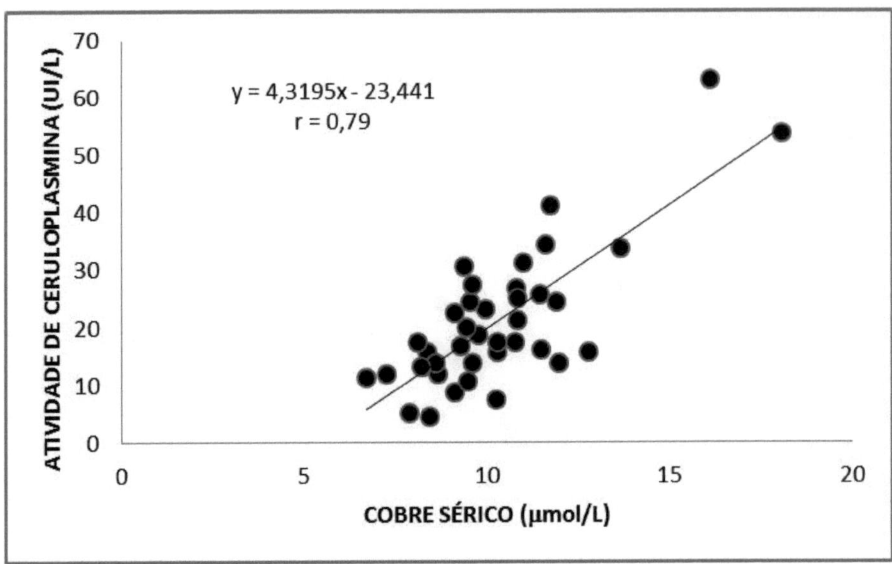

The analysis of the relationship between ceruloplasmin activity and serum copper in goats during the rainy season showed a high positive relationship (r = 0.61), and is expressed by the equation:

y = 0.0102x + 14.644

Graph 28 - Relationship between ceruloplasmin activity (IU/L) and serum copper (µmol/L) in goats during the rainy season.

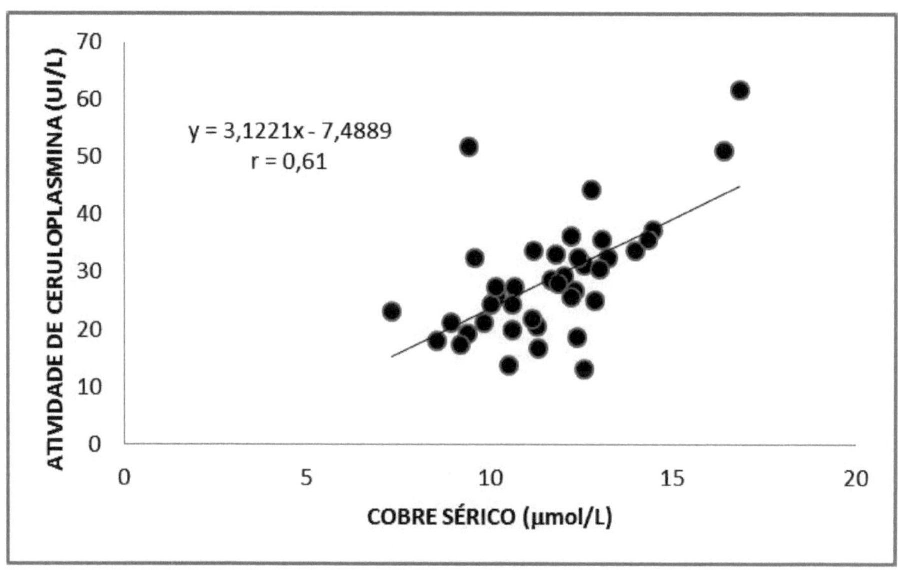

Analysis of the relationship between GGT activity and serum copper showed a low positive relationship (r = 0.19), expressed by the equation:

y = 1.2644x + 28.578

Graph 29 - Relationship between GGT activity (IU/L) and serum copper (µmol/L) in small ruminants from the Petrolina micro-region.

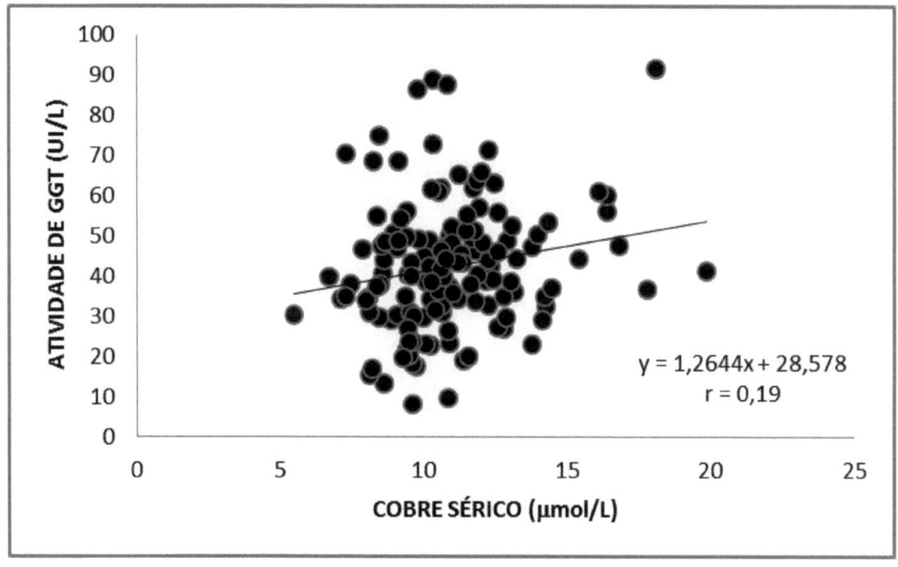

Analysis of the relationship between AST activity and serum copper showed a low negative relationship (r = 0.07), expressed by the equation:

y = -1.713x + 137.07

Graph 30 - Relationship between AST activity (IU/L) and serum copper (μmol/L) in small ruminants from the Petrolina micro-region.

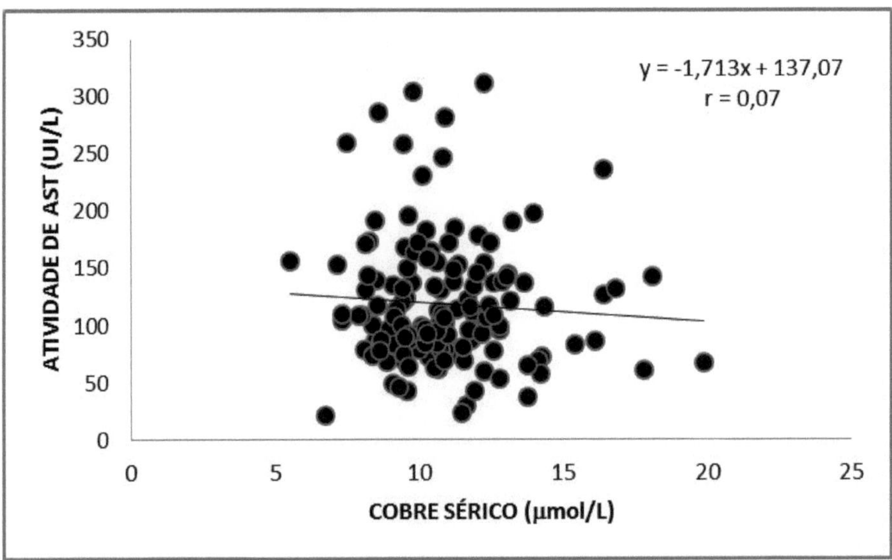

Analysis of the relationship between GGT activity and hepatic copper showed a low positive relationship (r = 0.05), expressed by the equation:

y = 0.0054x + 41.245

Graph 31 - Relationship between GGT activity (U I/L) and hepatic copper (μmol/L) in small ruminants from the Petrolina micro-region.

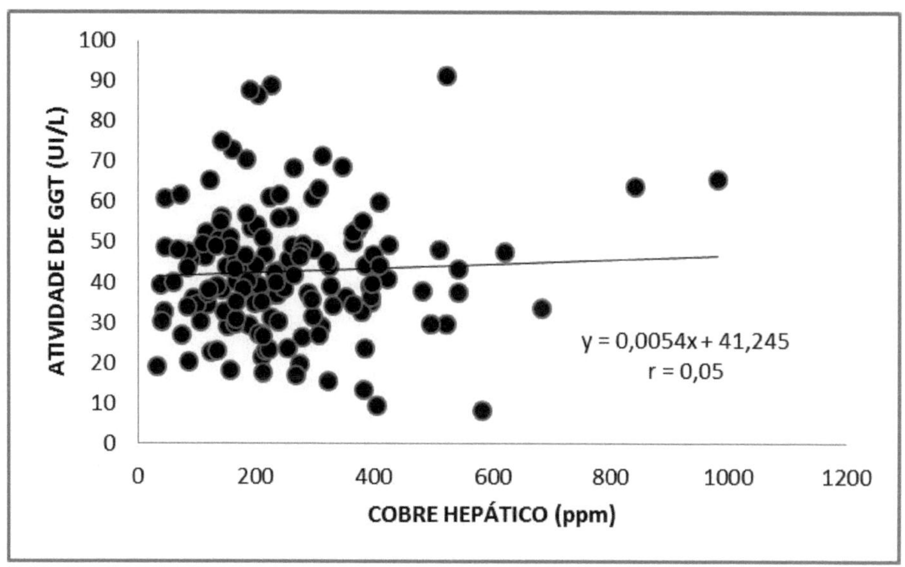

Analysis of the relationship between AST activity and liver copper showed a low positive relationship (r = 0.12), expressed by the equation:

y = 0.0489x + 107.38

Graph 32 - Relationship between AST activity (IU/L) and hepatic copper (μmol/L) in small ruminants from the Petrolina micro-region.

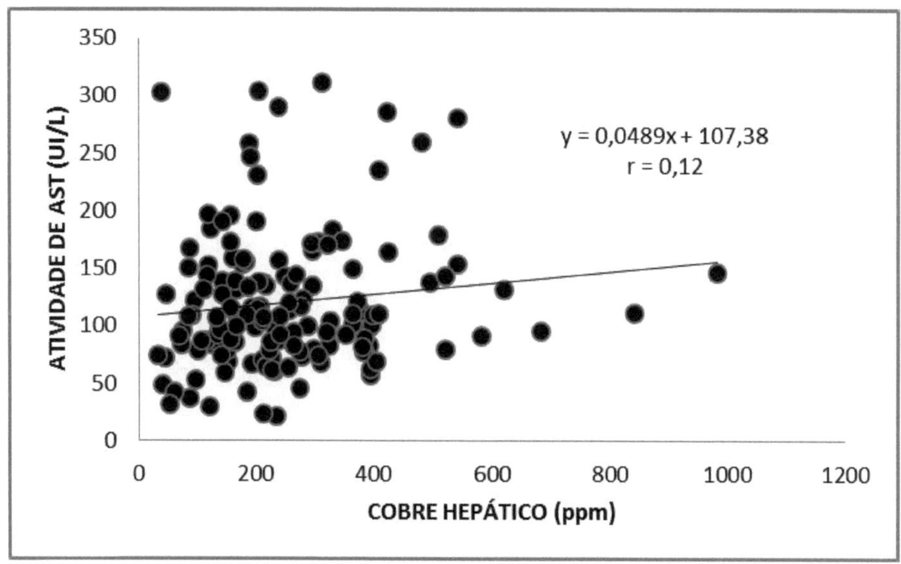

Discussion

This study showed that the animals slaughtered in the municipality of Petrolina, which come from the Petrolina micro-region, are raised in an extensive or semi-extensive system, without being fed concentrates. This fact has been shown by Maranhâo (2013), who states that the low productivity in the semi-arid northeast is due to this breeding system associated with the economic precariousness of the farmers. Silva et al. (2010) report that in the semi-arid region it is common practice for sheep farmers to use native pasture, based on the caatinga, as a source of food, which imposes serious restrictions on animal development during the dry season.

The drought that occurred in the Brazilian semi-arid region during this study, especially in the Petrolina micro-region, should be a factor to consider when evaluating the results of this work, as the average rainfall in Petrolina in September and October 2011 was 0.3 mm (historical average of 7 mm) and in March and April 2012 it was 2.0 mm (historical average of 75 mm) (EMBRAPA, 2013).

We found that the serum copper levels in sheep shown in Table 3 ranged from 9.8 to 10.7 μmol/L, with no difference between males and females or between the dry and rainy periods, and these results are within the reference values presented by Kaneko et al. (1997) (9.13 to 25.2 μmol/L), and close to the results reported by Marques et al. (2011), which show results obtained in the micro-region of Araripina, also located in the state of Pernambuco. However, the results obtained in this study are inferior to those published by Grace (1983), Van Ryssen and Bradifield (1992), Oregui and Bravo (1993) and Santos et al. (2006), and of these studies only Santos et al. (2006) was carried out in Brazil, more precisely in the municipality of Surubim-PE, located in the Agreste region of Pernambuco, with theoretically more favorable conditions for animal husbandry. In a study carried out in Mossoró-RN (SOUSA et al., 2012), average plasma copper values of 5.9 and 5.2 μmol/L were found in two farms in this municipality, where there was an outbreak of enzootic ataxia.

When we evaluate the results for the goats in this study, whose averages ranged from 10.2 to 12.6 μmol/L, we see that they are in line with the literature, where Marques (2010) shows values for goats of 11.37±2.57. Niekerk et al. (1990) shows values between 12.6 and 25.2 μmol/L and Solaiman et al. (2007) shows average values of 18.11 ± 0.63 μmol/L.

According to Suttle (2010), for small ruminants to show copper deficiency without apparent clinical manifestation, the serum value of this microelement needs to vary between 3 and 9 μmol/L, average values not found in this work. However, when we evaluated the individual data for each animal, eight goats and 17 sheep showed values within this range of inapparent copper deficiency.

When we analyzed the hepatic copper levels, we also found no difference between periods or species, with average values ranging from 217 to 295 ppm for sheep and 211 to 280 ppm for goats. These values are lower than those found by various authors: Jones et al. (1984) presented average values of 304 ppm; Oregui and Bravo (1993) reported that the average value of liver copper would be 500 ppm; Antonelli (2007) described average values of 328 ppm of copper in the liver as a parameter of normality in healthy sheep. Blood (1994) considers that normal values for liver copper occur from 200 ppm, while Grace (1983) considered values of 150 to 1,200 ppm of liver copper to be normal. There was also no variation between males and females, although Ortolani (2002) states that females may be more predisposed to copper accumulation, relating it to the action of oestradiol, which increases copper retention in the liver.

Although Suttle (1986) states that the determination of hepatic copper represents the accumulation of this element in the body rather than an indicator of deficiency, several authors have shown values lower than those found in this study and have determined them as apparent or inapparent copper deficiency. Marques (2010) suggested that values of 135 to 186 ppm indicate an apparent copper deficiency. Tokarnia et al. (1971) studied sheep with copper deficiency and found average hepatic copper values of 125 ppm, while Santos et al. (2006) showed that sheep and goats presented clinical signs of enzootic ataxia with values ranging from 19.4 to 140 ppm. In this study, although the average values were within normal parameters according to some authors, we obtained eight goats and 13 sheep with values lower than 110 ppm, which suggests that it is necessary to critically evaluate livestock and supplement with mineral mixtures animals raised in regions with food restrictions, such as the semi-arid region, because according to Peixoto et al. (2005), according to geographical location, time of year and type of feed, mineral supplementation should be indicated. NRC (2007) states that the requirements of goats in relation to copper in the diet is much higher than the requirements of sheep, considering the same weight and category, which presupposes a greater predisposition of goats in relation to the development of copper deficiency. This was suggested by Riet-Correa (2004) and confirmed by Santos et al. (2006) who found a higher incidence of enzootic ataxia in goats than in sheep. More studies are needed to better explain the causes of this predisposition.

As the serum and liver copper levels are within normal parameters according to various authors, this explains the low ratio between these two parameters. If there were a pronounced deficiency, or imminent intoxication, we would have a higher ratio, as shown by Antonelli (2007).

Another indicator of serum copper concentration is ceruloplasmin activity, which in this study showed a high ratio for goats and sheep in both periods, as shown in Graphs 25 to 28. Ceruloplasmin can be measured according to its serum concentration or serum oxidative activity. The serum oxidative activity of ceruloplasmin is related to the serum concentration of copper, i.e. a low concentration of this element is associated with lower ceruloplasmin activity.

Blakley and Hamilton (1985) found that the correlation between serum ceruloplasmin activity and serum copper concentration was 0.83 in cattle and 0.92 in sheep, and concluded that it can be used as an indicator of organic copper status in these species. This study corroborates that of Paynter (1982), who states that ceruloplasmin activity is a good indicator of copper concentration in serum and liver, recording values of 23.2 to 60.7 IU/L. While Kincaid (1986) stated that the correlation between serum ceruloplasmin and liver copper is low, around 0.35. In another study, serum ceruloplasmin concentration showed no significant correlation with plasma copper concentration (QUIROZ-ROCHA et al., 2003). As ceruloplasmin activity decreases with the drop in copper levels, cases of deficiency have higher correlation values. In this study, the ratio was not as high as in Blakley and Hamilton (1985), perhaps because the copper deficiency was not as pronounced.

Niekerk et al. (1990) showed zinc values below 12.2 µmol/L for both sheep and goats, which according to the authors indicates a marginal deficiency of this element. In our study, only female goats in the dry period showed average values lower than those described by Niekerk et al. (1990), suggesting a marginal deficiency of this element in this period. Suttle (2010) states that the lower limit of normality for serum zinc in sheep and goats is 10 µmol/L. In both cases, the female goats mentioned above would be within normal values, but very close to deficiency values. Marques (2010) found values ranging from 10.6 to 12.8 µmol/L. Van Ryssen and Bradifield (1992) found average values of 15.0 µmol/L for zinc in sheep kept on pasture, which was considered within normal range, but still below the average values found in our work, except for female goats in the dry period.

The hepatic zinc levels found in this study (104 to 133 ppm) were in line with those reported by Tokarnia et al. (1988), who stated that hepatic zinc levels ranged from 101 to 200 ppm, and slightly lower for some categories and periods than those found by Marques (2010), whose average values were 128.7 ppm, as well as by Antonelli (2007) in sheep, who reported normal values ranging from 120 to 138 ppm. Zinc is the main stimulator of hepatic metallothionein synthesis. According to López-Alonso et al. (2005), the higher the concentration of zinc in the liver, the higher the content of metallothionein in this organ (R^2 = 0.69). This compound is responsible for complexing with the copper stored in the organ to be subsequently excreted by the bile in the detoxification process.

Although he did not determine the levels of metallothionein, Minervino (2007) suggested that ruminants about to become intoxicated by copper begin to accumulate zinc in the liver in an attempt to increase copper detoxification. As in this study there were no large quantities of copper, there was probably no stimulus to store this element in large quantities, nor was there a high or medium relationship between hepatic copper accumulation and hepatic zinc accumulation.

The results obtained in this study, both for serum zinc and liver zinc, can be considered within the normal range according to some authors, but flirting with marginal values as they were very close to the lower limit of normality. As zinc absorption is influenced by the presence of antagonists such as copper, calcium and iron, and in this study relatively high iron values were found, this may have contributed to the decrease in zinc absorption. If the animal is deficient in zinc, reduced appetite and a selective appetite for protein and fat take precedence over carbohydrates, as well as resulting in dermatological abnormalities and bone and reproductive disorders (Suttle, 2010). It would therefore be interesting to evaluate the possible occurrence of infertility problems and low weight gain in these regions where low zinc levels have been proven.

Interesting data was obtained from serum iron, as sheep showed significantly higher values in the dry period (78.5 µmol/L) compared to the rainy period (51.2 µmol/L), as well as in relation to goats (45.4 µmol/L). According to Kaneko et al. (1997), the serum concentration of sheep ranges from 29.7 to 39.7 µmol/L, while Suttle (2010) considers the average value of 34.6±1.25 µmol/L for sheep and 17 to 36 µmol/L for goats to be normal, and Blood (1994) considers average values of 37.4 µmol/L to be normal. Analyzing the data obtained in this study, all the animals had serum values above those considered normal by the aforementioned authors. However, there is controversy in the literature, as Suttle (2010) states that sheep can have serum iron values ranging from 18.2 to 54.4 µmol/L, and thus only the dry period sheep had values higher than those considered to be within the normal range. Marques (2010) obtained values ranging from 25.06 to 35.58 µmol/L for serum iron in a region close to that of this study, a fact that can be explained by the more favorable rainfall conditions in the target municipalities of his study (Granito, Ouricuri and Araripina), in addition to the fact that there was considerably more rainfall at the time his study was conducted, increasing the supply of food. According to the aforementioned authors, the threshold for an animal to start developing iron deficiency is 29 μmol/L of serum iron, which is considered a risk factor for deficiency, while values above 39 μmol/L are indicative of excess serum iron.

The hepatic iron results in this study showed much higher values in sheep than in goats, being higher than the values found by Jones et al (1984) (138.8 ppm) and by Marques (2010) (156.1 to 210.5 ppm). Tokarnia et al. (1988) found values ranging from 181 to 380 ppm of hepatic iron. These higher concentrations in the serum and liver of sheep may be associated with the feeding habits of this species, which, according to Leite (2002), are classified as roughage users, preferring more dicotyledonous herbs and grasses, i.e. they graze closer to the ground. On the other hand, goats are classified as intermediate selectors, adapted to include a wide variety of plants in their diet, with an opportunistic and adaptive behavior to what the environment offers according to the availability of forage and the season of the year, preferring herbaceous dicotyledons and shoots and leaves of trees and shrubs (ARAÙJO FILHO et al., 1996; LEITE, 2002). Combined with the levels of iron available in the reference soils of Pernambuco, which are considered to be medium to high (OLIVEIRA; NASCIMENTO, 2006), we can suggest that the habit of eating undergrowth predisposes people to ingesting iron-containing soil, increasing the levels of this element in the body. Santos et al (2006) have already suggested this possibility, considering that during the dry season, pastures become scarcer, forcing animals to graze closer to the ground, which is rich in iron (8600 ppm), in addition to verifying that because it is a sandy soil, it covers the forage available to the animals in the form of dust, forcing the animals to ingest high amounts of iron.

Although Santos et al. (2006) and Suttle (2010) infer copper deficiency to iron excess, in this study the average copper levels were not deficient and there was a low ratio between iron and liver copper.

The serum molybdenum concentration showed surprising results, considering the extremely low values in the literature. Firstly, we found that 71.25% of the animals had serum molybdenum values of less than 0.05 μmol/L. It was not possible to determine the exact molybdenum content in these samples because the calibration curve of the optical plasma emission spectrometry apparatus did not allow lower values to be determined. These values are much lower than those found by Van Ryssen and Stielau (1981), who found average values of 0.63 μmol/L, Botha et al. (1995) who determined average values of 0.52 μmol/L, Pott et al. (1999) found an average serum molybdenum value of 0.10 μmol/L, Antonelli

(2007) found average serum values of 0.8 µmol/L, and Marques (2010) with values ranging from 0.28 to 0.32 µmol/L. Even when evaluating the serum values of the materials that could be read by the device, these were extremely low, ranging from 0.10 to 0.20 µmol/L, results that were only comparable to Pott et al. (1999).

With regard to hepatic molybdenum levels, we found that, except for the goats during the rainy season (0.8 ppm), the average values obtained varied between 2.4 and 3.3 ppm, which is in line with the results shown by various authors, despite the wide variation in the results presented. From the lowest hepatic molybdenum values found in the literature by Allen and Gawthorne (1986) with 1.8 ppm to 5.88 ppm with Pott et al. (1999). According to Suttle (2010), molybdenum levels in sandy soils, similar to those found at the site of this study, show extremely low levels of molybdenum, which is reflected in the content of this microelement in the vegetation. There is generally no concern about molybdenum deficiency, as there are no reports of adverse effects resulting from hypomolybdenosis (SUTTLE, 2010). It is therefore suggested that further studies with this microelement in animals be carried out concomitantly with the determination of its levels in soil and food in order to gain a better understanding of its status in the body, despite the fact that its main action is antagonism in relation to copper metabolism.

This antagonism is directly related to the presence of sulphur in the diet, where thiomolybdates are formed in the rumen, interfering with its absorption, as well as that of copper (SUTTLE, 2010). The very low values of molybdenum found in this study may explain the not very low levels of copper, which would be expected in animals raised extensively in the Serran region.

Without evaluating the presence of these microelements in the soil and pastures, it is not possible to state with certainty the origin of low or high values of any microelement, requiring further studies to explain the results found in this study. Even so, it is essential to analyze serum levels (homeostatic pool) and liver levels (stock) of microelements in animals, as little importance is given to some elements, such as iron in its ability to interfere with copper metabolism in extensively reared animals (HUMPHRIES et al., 1983). Therefore, these studies should be carried out together to provide a global view of copper metabolism together with the action of its antagonists (TOKARNIA et al., 1999).

This work, together with that carried out by Marques (2010), provides further insight into the status of these minerals in the Pernambuco state, making it possible to devise appropriate mineral supplementation strategies and improve productivity in this region of the state, where the extensive breeding system predominates among farmers.

The data obtained for GGT and AST, unlike studies related to copper intoxication, are not good parameters for estimating the accumulation of this element in the liver. Antonelli (2007) showed that GGT activity has 90% sensitivity and 100% specificity for estimating liver copper levels above 1000 ppm, while AST activity has 73% sensitivity and 100% specificity. This can be confirmed by the low relationship between liver copper content and the activity of these enzymes. Other indicators should therefore be investigated as tools for estimating copper accumulation in animals with normal or deficient copper levels.

Conclusions

Considering the average copper levels obtained, goats and sheep raised in the Petrolina micro-region do not present primary or secondary copper deficiency;

Considering the average iron values, sheep have very high levels of this element, suggesting a higher intake of this element due to the species' feeding habits;

It is suggested that hepatic copper accumulation in this region is not so low due to the region's low molybdenum content;

Ceruloplasmin activity is a good indicator of marginal serum copper status in small ruminants;

AST and GGT activities are not indicators of copper status for animals with low levels of this element in the liver.

REFERENCES

AGUILERA, J. F.; PRIETO, C.; FONOLLA, J. Protein and energy metabolism of lactating Grenadina goats. **British Journal of Nutrition**, v. 63, p. 165-175, 1990.

ALLEN, J. D.; GAWTHORNE, J. M. Involvement of the solid phase rumen digesta in the interactions between copper, molybdenum and sulphur in sheep. **British Journal of Nutrition**, v. 58, p. 265-276, 1987.

ANTONELLI, A. C. **Evaluation of the use of a mineral salt rich in molybdenum in the prevention of cumulative cupric intoxication in sheep**. 2007. 122 f. Thesis (Doctorate) - Faculty of Veterinary Medicine and Zootechny, University of Sao Paulo, Sao Paulo, 2007.

ARAÙJO FILHO, J. A.; SOUSA, F. B.; CARVALHO, F. C. Botanical and chemical composition of the diet of sheep and goats in combined grazing in the Inhamuns region, Cearà. **Revista da Sociedade Brasileira de Zootecnia**, v. 25, p. 383- 395, 1996.

ASHMEAD, H. D. Comparative intestinal absorption and sub-sequent metabolism of metal amino acid chelates and inorganic salts. In: ASHMEAD, H. D. **The Roles of Amino Acid Chelates in Animal Nutrition**. New Jersey: Noyes, 1993. P. 47-75.

BARONI, G; FONTEQUE, J, H; PAES, P. R. O; TAKAHIRA, R, K; KOHAYAGAWA, K; LOPES, R. S; LOPES, S. T. A; CROCCI, A. J. Serum calcium, phosphorus, sodium, potassium and total protein values in female Parda Alpina goats. **Ciência Rural**, v. 31, n.3, p. 435-438. 2001.

BARROS, N. N.; TEIXEIRA, L. B.; MORAES, E.; CANTO, A. C.; ITALIANO, E. C. Mineral contents in the soil-plant-animal complex of firm areas in Amazonas. **Comunicado Técnico,** n. 16, Manaus: Embrapa-UEPAE, 1981. 3 p.

BLAKLEY, B. R.; HAMILTON, D. L. Ceruloplasmin as an indicator of copper status in cattle and sheep. **Canadian Journal of Comparative Medicine**, v.49, p. 405-408, 1985.

BLOOD D. C. **Manual of Veterinary Medicine**. 1st ed. Philadelphia: Interamericana McGraw-Hill, 1994. 790 p.

BONDAN, E. F.; RIET-CORREA, F.; GIESTA, S. Hepatic levels of copper in cattle in the south of Rio Grande do Sul. **Pesquisa Veterinària Brasileira**, v. 11, n. 3/4, p. 75-80, 1991.

BOTHA, C. J.; GESWAN, G. E.; MINNAAR, P. P. Pharmacokinetics of ammonium tetrathiomolybdate following intravenous administration in sheep.

Journal of the South African Veterinary Association, v. 66, n. 1, p. 6-10, 1995.

BRAZIL. Ministry of Planning, Budget and Management. Brazilian Institute of Geography and Statistics - IBGE. **Municipal Livestock Production**. Brasilia, 2010.

BRAZIL. Ministry of Agrarian Development. Secretariat for Territorial Development. **Management Report**. Brasilia, 2011.

BRUM, P. A. R.; SOUSA, J. C.; COMASTRI FILHO, J. A.; ALMEIDA, I. L. Mineral deficiencies in cattle in the Paiaguâs sub-region, in the Pantanal of Mato Grosso. II. Copper, zinc, manganese and iron. **Pesquisa Agropecuâria Brasileira**, v. 22, n. 9/10, p. 1049-1060, 1987.

CARDOSO, E. C. **Nutriçâo mineral em bubalinos e bovinos nos campos do Marajó, estado do Parà: câcio, fósforo, cobre, cobalto, manganês, ferro e zinco**, 1997. 173 f. Thesis (Doctorate) - Federal University of Parà, Belém, 1997.

CAVALHEIRO A. C. L.; TRINDADE D. S. **Minerals for Cattle and Sheep Raised on Pasture**. Porto Alegre: Sagra-DC Luzzatto, 1992. 142 p.

CHAGAS A. C. S.; OLIVEIRA M. C. S.; FERNANDES L. B.; MACHADO R.; ESTEVES S. N.; SALES R. L.; BARIONI JUNIOR W. Control of worms, mineralization, reproduction and crossbreeding of sheep at Embrapa Pecuâria Sudeste. **Documentos 65**. Sao Carlos: Embrapa, 2007. 44 p.

CORAH, L. H.; IVES, S. The effects of essential trace minerals on reproduction in beef cattle. **Veterinary Clinics of North America: Food Animal Practice**, v. 7, n. 1, p. 41-57, 1991.

DAYRELL, M. S. Effect of mineral deficiencies on reproduction in cattle. **Documentos 50**. Coronel Pacheco: Embrapa, 1991, 18 p.

EMBRAPA. **Monthly rainfall (mm) at the Bebedouro Agrometeorological Station (Petrolina-pE 09°09'S 40°22'W).** Period 1975-2013. Petrolina, 2013. Available at: <http://www.cpatsa.embrapa.br:8080/servicos/dadosmet/ceb-chuva.html>.

Accessed on: May 15, 2013.

FERNANDES N. S.; SANTIAGO A. M. H. Levels of copper in pastures of the State of Mato Grosso. **Biological**, v. 38, n. 10, p. 358-360, 1972.

FERREIRA, M. B.; ANTONELLI, A. C.; ORTOLANI, E. L. Copper, selenium, zinc and sodium chloride poisoning. In: SPINOSA, H. S.; GÓRNIAK, S. L.;

PALERMO-NETO, J. **Toxicologia aplicada à Medicina Veterinària**. Barueri:

Manole, 2008. P. 665-697.

GENGELBACH G. P.; WARD J. D.; SPEARS J. W. Effect of dietary copper, iron, and molybdenum on growth and copper status of beef cows and calves. **Journal of Animal Science**, v. 72, n. 10, p. 2722-2727, 1994.

GONZALEZ, H. D.; BARCELLOS, J.; PATINO, H. O.; RIBEIRO, L. A. **Metabolic profile in ruminants: its use in nutrition and nutritional diseases**. Porto Alegre: UFRGS, 2000.

GRACE, N. D. Amounts and distribution of mineral elements associated with fleece-free empty body weight gains in the grazing sheep. **New Zealand Journal of Agricultural Research**, v. 26, p. 59-70, 1983.

GUEDES, K. M. R.; RIET-CORREA, F.; DANTAS, A. F.; SIMOES, S. V. D.; MIRANDA NETO, E. G.; NOBRE, V. M. T.; MEDEIROS, R. M. T. Diseases of the central nervous system in goats and sheep in the semi-arid region. **Pesquisa Veterinària Brasileira**, v. 27, n. 1, p. 29-38, 2007.

HERRICK, J. B. Minerals in animal health. In: ASHMEAD, H. D. **The roles of aminoacid chelates in animal nutrition**. New Jersey: Noyes Publication, 1993. p. 3-2.

HOWELL, J. M.; GOONERATNE, S. R. The pathology of copper toxicity in animals. **Copper in animals and man**. CRC Press, v. 2, p. 53-78, 1987.

HUMPHRIES, W. R. The influence of dietary iron and molybdenum on copper metabolism in calves. **British Journal of Nutrition**, v. 49, p. 77-86, 1983.

JONES H. B.; GOONERATNE, S. R.; HOWELL J. M. X-ray microanalysis of liver and kidney in copper loaded sheep with and without thiomolybdate administration. **Research in Veterinary Science**, v. 37, p. 273-282, 1984.

KANEKO, J. J.; HARVEY, J. W.; BRUSS, M. L. **Clinical biochemistry of domestic animals**. 5th ed. San Diego: Academic Press, 1997. 932 p.

KEGLEY, E. B., SPEARS, J. W. Biovariability of feed-grade copper sources (oxide, sulfate, or lysine) in growing cattle. **Journal of Animal Science**, v. 72, p. 2728-2734, 1994.

KINCAID, R.; GAY, C. C.; KRIEGER, R. I. Relationship of serum and plasma copper and ceruloplasmin concentrations of cattle and the effects of whole blood sample storage. **American Journal of Veterinary Research**, v. 47, p. 1157-1159, 1986.

LEITE, E. R. Dietary management of goats and sheep grazing in northeastern Brazil. **Ciência Animal**, v. 12, n. 2, p. 119-128, 2002.

LISBÔA, J. A. N.; KUCHEMBUCK, M. R. G.; KOHAYAGAWA, A.; BOMFIM, S. R. M.; SANTIAGO, A. M. H.; DUTRA, I. S. Results of clinical pathology and dosage of mineral elements in cattle affected by epizootic botulism in the State of Sao Paulo. **Pesquisa Veterinària Brasileira**, v. 16, n. 4, p. 91-97, 1996.

LITTLE, T. M.; HILLS, F. J. **Agricultural experimentation:** design and analysis. New York: John Wiley, 1978. 350 p.

LOPES, H. O. S.; FICHTNER, S. S.; JARDIM, E. C.; COSTA, C. P.; MARTINS JUNIOR, W. Copper and zinc contents in soil, forage and animal tissue samples from the Mato Grosso de Goiàs micro-region. **Arquivos da Escola de Veterinària da UFMG**, v. 32, n. 2, p. 151-159, 1980.

LÓPEZ-ALONSO, M; PRIETO, F.; MIRANDA, M.; CASTILLO, C.; HERNANDÉZ, J.; BENEDITO, J.L. The role of metallothionein and zinc in hepatic copper accumulation in cattle. **The Veterinary Journal**, v. 169, p. 262267, 2005.

LÓPEZ-ALONSO, M.; CRESPO, A.; MIRANDA, M.; CASTILLO, C.;

HERNANDEZ, J.; BENEDITO, J. L. Assessment of some blood parameters as potential markers of hepatic copper accumulation in cattle. **Journal of Veterinary Diagnostic Investigation**, v. 18, n. 1, p. 71-75, 2006.

MACHADO, C. H. **Use of tetrathiomolybdate in the treatment of experimental cupric intoxication in sheep:** clinical and toxicological evaluation, 1998. 138 f. Thesis (Doctorate) - Faculty of Veterinary Medicine and Zootechny, University of Sao Paulo, Sao Paulo, 1998.

MARANHÂO, R. L. A. **Dynamics of sheep production in Brazil from 1976 to 2010**, 2013. 42 f. Dissertation (Master's Degree) - Institute of Human Sciences, University of Brasilia, Brasilia, 2013.

MARQUES, A. P.; RIET-CORREA, F.; SOARES, M. P.; ORTOLANI, E. L.; GIULIODORI, M. J. Sudden deaths in cattle associated with copper deficiency. **Pesquisa Veterinària Brasileira**, v. 23, n. 1, p. 21-32, 2003.

MARQUES, A. V. S. **Copper content and its main antagonists in the liver and blood of sheep and goats raised in the state of Pernambuco**, 2010. 66 f. Dissertation (Master's Degree) - Department of Veterinary Medicine, Federal Rural University of Pernambuco, Recife, 2010.

MARQUES, A. V. S.; SOARES, P. C.; RIET-CORREA, F.; MOTA, I. O.; SILVA, T. L. A.; BORBA NETO, A V.; SOARES, F. A. P.; ALENCAR, S. P. Serum and liver levels of copper, iron, molybdenum and zinc in sheep and goats in the state of Pernambuco. **Pesquisa Veterinària Brasileira**, v. 31, n. 5, p. 398406, 2011.

MASSAD , E.; MENEZES, R. X.; SILVEIRA, P. S. P.; ORTEGA, N. R. S. **Métodos quantitativos em medicina**. Barueri: Manole, 2004. 561 p.

MAXIE, M. G. **Jubb, Kennedy and Palmer's Pathology of Domestic Animals**. 5. ed. St. Louis: Elsevier, 2007. 2340 p.

MAYNARD, L. A. **Nutriçâo animal**. 3 ed. Rio de Janeiro: Freitas Bastos, 1984. p. 260-280.

McDOWELL, L. R. **Minerals in Animal and Human Nutrition**. New York: Academic Press, 1992. 524 p.

McDOWELL, L. R. **Minerals for grazing ruminants in tropical regions, emphasizing Brazil**. 3. ed. Gainesville: University Press, 1999. 292 p.

MENDONÇA JÛNIOR, A. F.; BRAGA, A. P.; RODRIGUES, A. P. M. S.; SALES, L. E. M.; MESQUITA, H. C. Minerals: importance of use in ruminant diets. **Agropecuâria Cientifica no Semiàrido**, v. 7, n. 1, p. 1-13, 2011.

MILES, P. H.; WILKINSON, N. S.; McDOWELL, L. R. Analysis of Minerals for Animal Nutrition Research. 3. ed. Florida: University Press, 2001. 117 p.

MILLS, C. F. Biochemical and physiological indicators of mineral status in animals: copper, cobalt and zinc. **Journal Animal Science**, v. 65, n. 6, p. 1702-1711, 1987.

MINERVINO, A. H. H. **Comparative study of the susceptibility of cattle and buffalo to cumulative cupric intoxication.** 2007. 99 p. Dissertaçâo (Master's Degree) - Faculty of Veterinary Medicine and Zootechny, University of Sâo Paulo, Sâo Paulo, 2007.

MINITAB. **The student edition of MINITAB statistical software adapted for education**: 13.0 release; user's manual. New York: Wesley, 2000. 624 p.

MONDAL M. K.; BISWAS P. Different Sources and Levels of Copper Supplementation on Performance and Nutrient Utilization of Castrated Black Bengal (*Capra hircus*) Kids Diet. **Asian Australasian Journal of Animal Science**, v. 20, n. 7, p. 1067-1075, 2007.

MORAES S. S.; TOKARNIA C. H.; DOBEREINER J. Deficiencies and imbalances of microelements in cattle and sheep in some regions of Brazil. **Pesquisa Veterinària Brasileira**, v. 19, n. 1, p. 19-33, 1999.

MORAIS, M. G., RANGEL, J. M., MADUREIRA, J. S., SILVEIRA, A. C. Seasonal variation in clinical biochemistry of ring-bred cows under continuous grazing of Brachiaria decumbens. **Arquivo Brasileiro de Medicina Veterinària e Zootecnia**, v. 52, n. 2, p. 98-104, 2000.

NATIONAL RESEARCH COUNCIL - NRC. COMMITTEE ON THE NUTRIENT REQUIREMENTS OF SMALL RUMINANTS. **Nutrient Requirements of Small Ruminants: Sheep, Goats, Cervids, and New World Camelids**. Washington, D.C.: National Academy Press, 2007. 384 p.

NIEKERK, F. E. van; CLOETE, S. W. P.; BARNARD, S. A.; HEINE, E. W. P. Plasma copper, zinc and blood selenium concentrations of sheep, goats and cattle. **South African Journal of Animal Science**, v. 20, n. 3, p. 144-147, 1990.

OLIVEIRA, A. B.; NASCIMENTO, W. A. Forms of manganese and iron in reference soils of Pernambuco. **Revista Brasileira de Ciência do Solo**, v. 30, n. 1, p. 99-110, 2006.

OREGUI, L. M.; BRAVO, M. V. Copper, functions and needs. In: OREGUI L. M. **Copper-related pathology**: Deficiencias e intoxicaciones. 1. ed. Madrid: Luzans Ediciones, 1993. P. 9-22.

ORTOLANI, E. L. Macro and microelements. In: SPINOSA, H. S.; GÓRNIAK, S. L.; BERNARDI, M. M. **Farmacologia aplicada à medicina veterinària**. 3. ed. Rio de Janeiro: Guanabara Koogan, 2002. P. 641-651.

ORTOLANI, E. L. Cumulative copper poisoning in sheep. In: CONGRESSO BRASILEIRO DE BUIATRIA, 5, 2003, Salvador. **Book of Abstracts and Lectures**. Salvador: Venture, 2003. P. 113-114.

PAYNTER, D. I. Differences between serum and plasma ceruloplasmin activities and copper concentrations: investigation of possible contributing factors. **Australian Journal of Biological Science**, v. 35, p 353-361, 1982.

PEIXOTO, P. V.; MALAFAIA, P.; BARBOSA, J. D.; TOKARNIA, C. H. Principios de suplementaçâo mineral em ruminantes. **Pesquisa Veterinària Brasileira**, v. 25, n. 3, p. 195-200, 2005.

POTT, E. B.; ALMEIDA, I. L.; BRUM, P. A. R.; COMASTRI FILHO, J. A.; POTT, A.; DYNIA, J. E. Mineral nutrition of beef cattle in the Pantanal of Mato Grosso. 2. Micronutrients in Nhecolândia (central part). **Pesquisa Agropecuària Brasileira**, v. 24, n. 1, p. 109-126, 1989.

POTT E. B.; HENRY P. R.; ZANETTI M. A.; RAO P. V.; HINDERBERGER E. J.; AMMERMAN C. B. Effetcs of hight molybdenum concentration and duration of feeding time on molybdenum and copper metabolism in sheep. **Animal Feed Science and Technology**, v. 79, p. 93-105, 1999.

QUIROZ-ROCHA, G. F.; BOUDA, J. OCHOA, L. N.; FERREYRA, C. S.; MATA, D. A. C. Comparison of serum ceruloplasmin and copper with liver copper as indicators of body copper status in discarded cows. **Veterinaria México**, v. 34, n. 2, p. 143-148, 2003.

RADOSTITS, O. M.; GAY, C. C.; HINCHCLIFF, K. W.; CONSTABLE, P. D. **Veterinary Medicine:** a textbook of the diseases of cattle, horses, sheep, pigs, and goats. 10. ed. Philadelphia: Saunders Elsevier, 2007. 2156 p.

RIET-CORREA, F.; BONDAN, E. F.; MENDEZ, M. C.; MORAES, S. S.;

CONCEPCIÓN M. R. Effect of copper supplementation and diseases associated with copper deficiency in cattle in Rio Grande do Sul. **Pesquisa Veterinària Brasileira**, v. 13, n. 3/4, p. 45-49, 1993.

RIET-CORREA, F. Mineral supplementation in small ruminants in the semi-arid region. **Ciência Veterinària nos Trópicos**, v. 7, n. 2/3, p. 112-130, 2004.

RIET-CORREA, F.; SCHILD, A. L.; MÉNDEZ, M. C.; LEMOS, R. A. A. **Diseases of Ruminants and Equines**. 2. ed. Sâo Paulo: Varela, 2006. V. 2, 574 p.

SAMPAIO, I. B. M. **Estatistica aplicada à experimentaçâo animal**. Belo Horizonte: Fundaçâo de Ensino e Pesquisa em Medicina Veterinària e Zootecnia, 1998. 221 p.

SANTOS, N. V. M.; SARKIS, J. E. S.; GUERRA, J. L.; MAIORKA, P. C.; HORTELANI, M. A.; SILVA, F. F.; ORTOLANI, E. L. Epidemiological, clinical, anatomopathological and etiological evaluation of outbreaks of ataxia in kids and lambs. **Ciência Rural**, v. 36, n. 4, p. 1207-1213, 2006.

SCHOSINSKY, K. H.; LEHMANN, H. P.; BEELER, M. F. Measurement of ceruloplasmin from its oxidase activity in serum by use of dianisidine dihydrochloride. **Clinical Chemistry**, v. 20, n. 12, p. 1556-1563, 1974.

SIEGEL, S. **Nonparametric Statistics**. Sâo Paulo: McGraw-Hill, 1975. 350 p.

SILVA, N. V. S.; COSTA, R. G.; FREITAS, C. R. G.; GALINDO, M. C. T.;

SILVA, L. S. Sheep feeding in semi-arid regions of Brazil. **Acta Veterinaria Brasilica**, v. 4, n. 4, p. 233-241, 2010.

SKINNER, J. G. International standardization of acute phase proteins. Special Report. **Veterinary Clinical Pathology**, v. 30, n. 1, p. 2-7, 2001.

SNEDCOR, G. W.; COCHRAN, W. G. **Statistical methods**. 6. ed. Ames: Iowa State University Press, 1967. 593 p.

SOLAIMAN S. G.; SHOEMAKER C. E.; JONES W. R.; KERTH C. R. The effects of high levels of supplemental copper on the serum lipid profile, carcass traits, and carcass composition of goat kids. **Journal of Animal Science**, v. 84, p. 171-177, 2006.

SOLAIMAN, T. J.; CRAIG, J. R.; REDDY, G.; SHOEMAKER, C. E. Effect of high levels of Cu supplement on growth performance, rumen fermentation, and immune responses in goat kids. **Small Ruminant Research**, v. 69, n. 1, p. 115123, 2007.

SOUSA, I. K. F.; MINERVINO, A. H. H.; SOUSA, R. S.; CHAVES, D. F.; SOARES, H. S.; BARROS, I. O.; ARAÙJO, C. A. S. C.; BARRÊTO JÙNIOR, R.

A.; ORTOLANI, E. L. Copper deficiency in sheep with high liver iron accumulation. **Veterinary Medicine International**, v. 2012, art. 207950, p. 1-4, 2012.

SOUSA, J. C.; CONRAD, J. H.; McDOWELL, L. R.; AMMERMAN, C. B.; BLUE, W. G. Interrelationships between minerals in soil, forage and animal tissue. 2.

Copper and molybdenum. **Pesquisa Agropecuâria Brasileira**, v. 15, n. 3, p. 335 341, 1980.

SOUSA, J. C. Aspectos da suplementaçâo mineral de bovinos de corte. **Technical circular - EMBRAPA**, n. 5, p. 50, 1981.

SOUSA, J. C., NICODEMO, M. L. F.; DARSIE, G. Mineral deficiencies in cattle in Roraima, Brazil. V. Copper and molybdenum. **Pesquisa Agropecuâria Brasileira**, v. 24, n. 12, p. 1547-1554, 1989.

SUTTLE N. F. Copper deficiency in ruminants: recent developments. **Veterinary Records**, v. 119, n. 21, p. 519-522, 1986.

SUTTLE, N. F. **Mineral Nutrition of Livestock**. 4th ed. Oxfordshire: CABI Publishing, 2010. 587 p.

TEBALDI, F. L. H.; SILVA, J. F. C.; VASQUEZ, H. M.; THIEBAUT, J. T. L. Mineral composition of pastures in the north and northwest regions of the State of Rio de Janeiro. 2. Manganese, iron, zinc, copper, cobalt, molybdenum and lead. **Revista Brasileira de Zootecnia**, v. 29, n. 2, p. 616-629, 2000.

TOKARNIA, C. H.; CANELLA C. F. C.; DOBEREINER, J. Copper deficiency in cattle in the Parnaiba River Delta, in the states of Piaui and Maranhao.

Archives of the Institute of Animal Biology, v. 3, p. 25-37, 1960.

TOKARNIA, C. H.; CANELLA C. F. C.; GUIMARAES J. A.; DOBEREINER, J. Copper and cobalt deficiency in cattle and sheep in the Northeast and North of Brazil. **Pesquisa Agropecuâria Brasileira**, v. 3, p. 351-360, 1968.

TOKARNIA, C. H.; DOBEREINER, J.; CANELLA C. F. C.; GUIMARAES J. A. Enzootic ataxia in lambs in Piaui. **Pesquisa Agropecuâria Brasileira**, v. 1, p. 375-382, 1966.

TOKARNIA, C. H.; DOBEREINER, J.; MORAES, S. S. Current situation and perspectives of research on mineral nutrition in cattle in Brazil. **Pesquisa Veterinària Brasileira**, v. 8, n. 1/2, p. 1-16, 1988.

TOKARNIA, C. H.; DOBEREINER, J.; MORAES, S. S.; PEIXOTO, P. V. Mineral deficiencies and imbalances in cattle and sheep - review of studies carried out in Brazil from 1987 to 1998. **Pesquisa Veterinària Brasileira**, v. 19, n. 2, p. 47-62, 1999.

TOKARNIA, C. H.; DOBEREINER, J.; PEIXOTO, P. V. Mineral deficiencies in farm animals, mainly cattle. **Pesquisa Veterinària Brasileira**, v. 20, n. 3, p.127-138, 2000.

TOKARNIA, C. H.; GUIMARAES J. A.; CANELLA C. F. C.; DOBEREINER, J. Copper and cobalt deficiency in cattle and sheep in some regions of Brazil. **Pesquisa Agropecuâria Brasileira**, v. 6, p. 61-77, 1971.

TRINDADE, D. S.; CAVALHEIRO, A. C. L.; ARNT, L. M. Concentrations of copper, zinc and sulphur in pastures of Rio Grande do Sul. **Revista da Sociedade Brasileira de Zootecnia**, v. 19, p. 489-497, 1990.

VAN RYSSEN, J. B.; STIELAU, W. J. Effect of different levels of dietary molybdenum on copper and Mo metabolism in sheep fed on high levels of Cu. **British Journal of Nutrition**, v. 45, p. 203-210, 1981.

VAN RYSSEN, J. B, BRADFIELD, G. D. An assessment of the selenium, copper and zinc status of sheep on cultivated pastures in the Natal Midlands. **Journal of South African Veterinary Association**, v. 63, n. 4, p. 156-161, 1992.

VASQUEZ, E. F. A.; HERRERA, A. P. N.; SANTIAGO, G. S. Interaction between copper, molybdenum and sulphur in ruminants. **Ciência Rural**, v. 31, n. 6, p. 1101-1106, 2001.

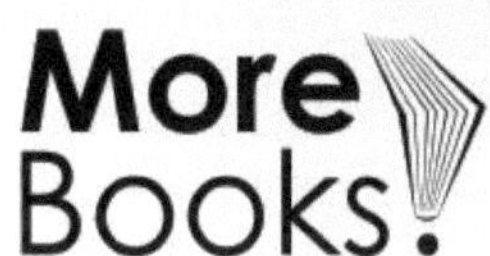

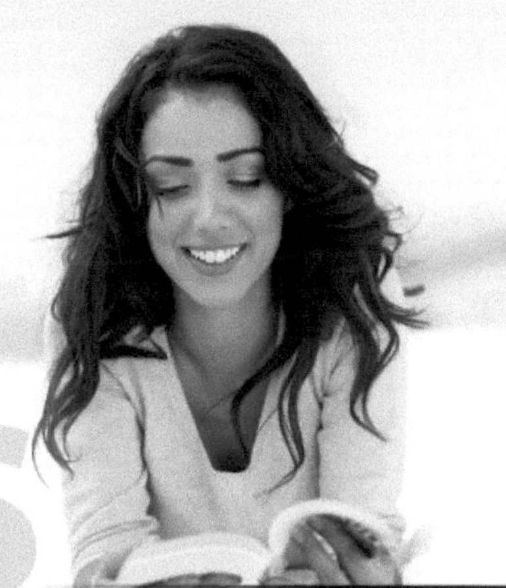

yes

I want morebooks!

Buy your books fast and straightforward online - at one of world's fastest growing online book stores! Environmentally sound due to Print-on-Demand technologies.

Buy your books online at

www.morebooks.shop

Kaufen Sie Ihre Bücher schnell und unkompliziert online – auf einer der am schnellsten wachsenden Buchhandelsplattformen weltweit! Dank Print-On-Demand umwelt- und ressourcenschonend produzi ert.

Bücher schneller online kaufen

www.morebooks.shop

info@omniscriptum.com
www.omniscriptum.com

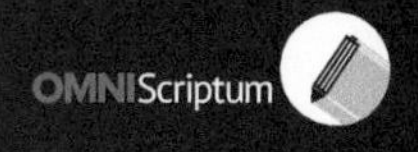

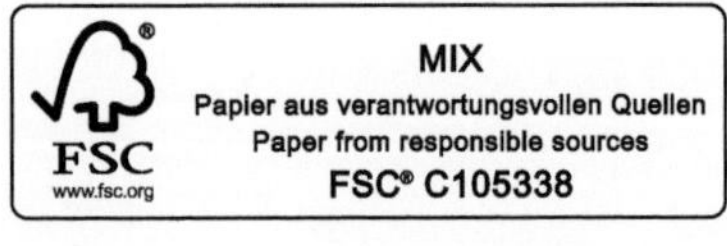

Printed by Books on Demand GmbH, Norderstedt / Germany